Radiation Medicine Rounds

Charles R. Thomas, Jr., MD

Editor-in-Chief

Professor and Chair
Department of Radiation Medicine
Professor, Division of Hematology/Oncology
Department of Medicine
Knight Cancer Institute
Oregon Health Sciences University
Portland, Oregon

Editorial Board

Forthcoming Issues

Prostate Cancer
Srinivasan Vijayakumar, MD, DMRT, FACR and Allen Chen, MD
Guest Editors

Head and Neck Cancer
Dwight E. Heron, MD and Roy Tishler, MD, PhD
Guest Editors

Radiation Medicine Rounds

VOLUME 1, ISSUE 3

Proton Therapy

Guest Editor

James M. Metz, MD

Associate Professor
Vice Chair, Clinical Division
Department of Radiation Oncology
Hospital of the University of Pennsylvania
Philadelphia, Pennsylvania

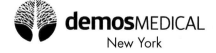

demosMEDICAL

New York

Acquisitions Editor: Richard Winters
Cover Design: Joe Tenerelli
Compositor: NewGen Imaging
Printer: Hamilton Printing

Visit our website at www.demosmedpub.com

Radiation Medicine Rounds is published three times a year by Demos Medical Publishing.

Business Office. All business correspondence including subscriptions, renewals, and address changes should be sent to Demos Medical Publishing, 11 West 42nd Street, 15th Floor, New York, NY, 10036.

The ideas and opinions expressed in *Radiation Medicine Rounds* do not necessarily reflect those of the Publisher. The Publisher does not assume any responsibility for any injury and/or damage to persons or property arising out of or related to any use of the material contained in this periodical. The reader is advised to check the appropriate medical literature and the product information currently provided by the manufacturer of each drug to be administered to verify the dosage, the method and duration of administration, or contraindications. It is the responsibility of the treating physician or other health care professional relying on independent experience and knowledge of the patient, to determine drug dosages and the best treatment for the patient. Mention of any product in this issue should not be construed as endorsement by the contributors, editors, or the Publisher of the product or manufacturer's claims.

ISSN: 2151-4208
ISBN: 978-1-617050-44-2

Library of Congress Cataloging-in-Publication Data

Proton therapy / guest editor, James M. Metz.
    p. ; cm. — (Radiation medicine rounds, ISSN 2151-4208 ; v. 1, issue 3)
  Includes bibliographical records and index.
  ISBN 978-1-936287-15-4 — ISBN 978-1-617050-44-2
  1. Cancer—Radiotherapy. 2. Protons—Therapeutic use. I. Metz, James M. II. Series: Radiation medicine rounds;
  v. 1, issue 3. 2151-4208
  [DNLM: 1. Protons—therapeutic use. 2. Radiotherapy—methods. 3. Neoplasms—radiotherapy. WN 250]

  RC271.R3P765 2010
  616.99'40642—dc22

                                                                                          2010044172

Reprints. For copies of 100 or more of articles in this publication, please contact Reina Santana, Special Sales Manager.

Special discounts on bulk quantities of Demos Medical Publishing books are available to corporations, professional associations, pharmaceutical companies, health care organizations, and other qualifying groups. For details, please contact:

Reina Santana, Special Sales Manager
Demos Medical Publishing
11 W. 42nd Street
New York, NY 10036
Phone: 800–532–8663 or 212–683–0072
Fax: 212–941–7842
E-mail: rsantana@demosmedpub.com

Made in the United States of America
10 11 12   13   14   5 4 3 2 1

Contents

Foreword

Radiation Medicine Rounds is a hard cover periodical published three times a year that is designed to provide an up-to-date review of defined radiation medicine topics of interest to clinicians and scientists who are involved in the care of patients receiving radiotherapy. It is intended to serve as both a reference and instructional tool by students, housestaff, fellows, practicing clinicians, medical physicists, cancer biologists, radiobiologists, and interdisciplinary colleagues throughout the oncology spectrum.

For the current issue, *Proton Therapy*, Guest Editor Dr. James Metz has overseen the development of timely articles on one of the most discussed technological advances in the delivery of modern radiotherapy. To his credit and that of the authors, this publication presents a balanced presentation of what we know and what has yet to be proven in the use of particle therapy. The contributions include highly desired discussions on the multidimensional aspect of concept development and eventual execution of a strategy that results in an active program, whether based in a traditional academic institution or in select community settings. Those who are committed to acquiring particle therapy and, more important, those who are undecided as to the overall merits of this expensive technology, will benefit from the articles within this book.

CHARLES R. THOMAS, JR.
Editor-in-Chief

Preface

Proton therapy is one of the most talked about areas in radiation oncology. There are strong opinions both within and outside the field on the use of proton therapy. We are experiencing rapid growth of new clinical centers, development of new technology to increase access, but also demands to show the value of this treatment modality. The articles within this issue address many of the topics under discussion today and emphasize the latest data from experts in the field. Although not every topic could be addressed in this book, we have tried to include many of the controversial issues and the most promising treatment areas for protons.

This issue starts with an overview of the physics and radiobiology of proton therapy and includes some of the important new developments on the horizon. Many of the major disease sites where proton therapy is commonly used are addressed in this volume with analysis of the evidence for treatment of these areas. An update on the use of proton therapy for lung cancer and thoracic tumors addresses important issues such as organ motion in proton therapy. The evidence for utilization of proton therapy in prostate cancer is dissected with a thorough discussion. The available data for treating tumors located in the brain and base of skull are discussed in another article. There is also a thorough review of the current evidence for treating pediatric malignancies with proton therapy.

This issue also reviews other unique areas in proton therapy, which are timely to the discussions around this technology. There is an intriguing article of the role of clinical trials in proton therapy that summarizes and dissects some of the most controversial arguments about protons. An additional article reviews the expansion of proton therapy into the community setting. And finally, we have included an article on the issues one must consider from a business perspective in building a proton therapy center.

I am sure that you will find this issue both engaging and timely.

James M. Metz, MD

Contributors

Christopher G. Ainsley, PhD
Assistant Professor
Department of Radiation Oncology
University of Pennsylvania
Philadelphia, Pennsylvania

Michelle Alonso-Basanta, MD, PhD
Helene Blum Assistant Professor
Department of Radiation Oncology
University of Pennsylvania Health System
Philadelphia, Pennsylvania

Keith A. Cengel, MD, PhD
Assistant Professor
Department of Radiation Oncology
University of Pennsylvania
Philadelphia, Pennsylvania

Joe Y. Chang, MD, PhD
Associate Professor and Clinical Service Chief
Department of Radiation Oncology
The University of Texas MD Anderson Cancer Center
Houston, Texas

John P. Christodouleas, MD, MPH
Assistant Professor
Department of Radiation Oncology
University of Pennsylvania School of Medicine
Philadelphia, Pennsylvania

Michael J. Eblan, BS
Pre-Doctoral Researcher
Department of Radiation Oncology
University of Pennsylvania
Philadelphia, Pennsylvania

Stephen M. Hahn, MD
Henry K. Pancoast Professor and Chair
Department of Radiation Oncology
University of Pennsylvania School of Medicine
Philadelphia, Pennsylvania

Ritsuko Komaki, MD
Professor
Department of Radiation Oncology
The University of Texas MD Anderson Cancer Center
Houston, Texas

Sameer Keole, MD
Adjunct Assistant Professor
Department of Radiation Oncology
Oklahoma University Health Science Center
Oklahoma City, Oklahoma

Sean M. McBride, MD
Resident
Department of Radiation Oncology
Massachusetts General Hospital
Boston, Massachusetts

James E. McDonough, PhD
Clinical Associate Professor
Department of Radiation Oncology
University of Pennsylvania
Philadelphia, Pennsylvania

Lynda J. Mischel
Chief Operating Officer
Department of Radiation Oncology
University of Pennsylvania Health System
Philadelphia, Pennsylvania

Carl J. Rossi, Jr., MD
Associate Professor
Department of Radiation Oncology
Loma Linda University Medical Center
Loma Linda, California

Torunn I. Yock, MD, MCH
Assistant Professor
Department of Radiation Oncology
Massachusetts General Hospital
Boston, Massachusetts

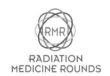

RADIATION
MEDICINE ROUNDS

Physics Considerations in Proton Therapy

Christopher G. Ainsley* and James E. McDonough
University of Pennsylvania, Philadelphia, PA

■ ABSTRACT

Despite being demonstrated for the first time over half a century ago, proton therapy has only really become a viable treatment option for patients suffering from cancer in the past 20 years. This chapter presents the reasons for the recent explosion of interest in proton therapy, together with some of the challenges faced in the implementation of clinical treatment systems. To begin, it describes the fundamental advantages that proton therapy offers over conventional x-ray-based approaches, recounts the key historical developments that have taken place enabling it to enter the mainstream of radiation oncology, and introduces the physics that underlies its effectiveness. Moving on, it compares alternative methods of generating clinically useful proton beams, evaluates the relative merits of various delivery techniques, and reviews issues of importance in planning proton therapy treatments. The chapter concludes with a view to the future.

Keywords: proton therapy physics, history, rationale, accelerators, scatterings, scanning, treatment planning

■ INTRODUCTION

Rationale

The goal of radiation therapy is to induce tumor-cell death by inflicting irreparable damage to DNA. In principle, therefore, success in tumor control is simply a matter of delivering an adequate dose of radiation to the target region. In practice, however, this may not always be possible because of the associated radiation-induced morbidity incurred by normal, healthy tissues.

External-beam radiation therapy is administered conventionally by beams of megavoltage x-ray photons. Unfortunately, the physical characteristics of photon beams do not lend themselves ideally to the task at hand. Beyond a short dose build-up, the depth of which increases from approximately 0.5 cm for a 1 MV beam to approximately 3.0 cm

*Corresponding author, Department of Radiation Oncology, Hospital of the University of Pennsylvania, 2 Donner Building, 3400 Spruce Street, Philadelphia, PA 19104

E-mail address: ainsley@uphs.upenn.edu

Radiation Medicine Rounds 1:3 (2010) 415–440.
DOI: 10.5003/2151–4208.1.3.415

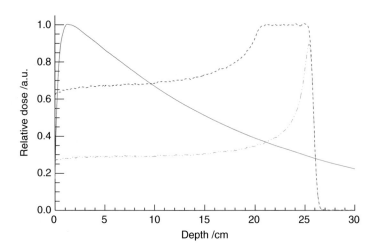

FIGURE 1

Comparison of the depth–dose distributions for a 6 MV photon beam (solid line) and an unmodulated (pristine) and modulated (SOBP) 200 MeV proton beam (dot-dashed and dashed lines, respectively).

for a 15 MV beam, the rate of energy deposition decreases approximately exponentially with depth in tissue (Figure 1). Any given beam thus penetrates the entire body, depositing dose all the way along its path, with the largest deposition occurring near the surface. Consequently, the delivery of a dose of radiation to a deep-seated tumor with a single x-ray beam requires the irradiation of tissues both proximal and distal to the target, with the proximal tissue invariably receiving a dose higher than the target itself. This effect can be mitigated to some extent, while improving dose homogeneity throughout the target, by designing treatment plans that direct beams at the target from multiple angles. The price to pay in so doing, though, is the low-dose irradiation of a higher volume of normal tissues.

One of the primary concerns with intensity-modulated radiation therapy (IMRT)—the most conformal x-ray-beam technique available today—is the undesirably, and unavoidably, high integral dose delivered to the patient. The exposure of a high volume of normal tissue to low-dose radiation

has the potential, over 20 to 30 years, to lead to the development of secondary malignancies. Though this is a valid concern among the population of cancer survivors at large, it is especially important in the case of pediatric patients cured of disease, who may live long enough to allow such effects to manifest over time. In this group of patients, much can be gained by sparing the many normal tissues that are still undergoing development (1).

By contrast, the physical characteristics of proton beams are ostensibly rather better suited for radiotherapeutic use (Figure 1). Protons traveling through tissue lose energy continuously and at an ever-increasing rate. The rate of energy loss reaches a maximum in the last few millimeters of the proton range and is termed the "Bragg peak" after William H. Bragg, who, in 1903, was the first to observe this phenomenon. The depth of the Bragg peak is a function of the initial energy of the proton beam: the higher this energy, the deeper the peak. A proton beam with an initial energy of 250 MeV is sufficient to penetrate a thickness of tissue greater than half the cross-sectional diameter of a typical human body. By appropriate selection of beam angle and incident energy, it is thus possible to deliver the peak dose precisely to the site of disease, no matter its location, while delivering essentially no dose to all tissues beyond. Furthermore, the energy and intensity of the beam can be varied in order to modify the Bragg peak, translating it throughout the longitudinal extent of the tumor. By generating a "spread-out Bragg peak" (SOBP) from a "pristine peak" in this way, and unlike a single x-ray beam, even a solitary proton beam has the potential to deliver a uniform dose to a target volume (Figure 1).

The enhanced target conformality afforded by a proton, as opposed to a photon, depth–dose distribution results in an overall smaller volume of irradiated normal tissue and a lower integral dose (Figure 2) (2). Not only does this reduce the risk of second malignancies but it also furnishes the possibilities of tumor dose escalation and reduced toxicity when used in combination with chemotherapy, both of which increase the probability of tumor control by comparison with x-ray therapy. It also presents the opportunity for hypofractionation, which would reduce the duration of a treatment course.

History

The potential therapeutic use of protons was first recognized in 1946 by Robert R. Wilson (3), based on the physical aspects of their dose distribution in matter. At that time, he also proposed several of the concepts that are in use today in proton therapy centers around the world, including the range modulator wheel—alluded to previously and described further in the Passive Scattering section—as a means of energy-modulating the proton beam in order to achieve a uniform dose over an extended target volume, and ionization chambers for use in monitoring the beam and to facilitate dose calibration.

The first use of proton beams for the treatment of human patients took place in the mid-1950s at the University of California Lawrence Berkeley Laboratory (LBL); not by coincidence,

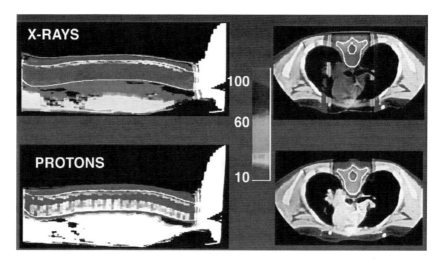

FIGURE 2

Comparison of dose distributions for spinal fields used to treat medulloblastoma, planned alternatively with photons (upper) and protons (lower). The proton treatment avoids an exit dose and thereby spares the contents of the mediastinum and anterior chest from irradiation.

TABLE 1
Worldwide proton therapy facilities currently or previously in operation

Location	Country	First treatment	Last treatment	Patient total	Date of total	Comment
Berkeley	CA, USA	1954	1957	30	-	
Uppsala (1)	Sweden	1957	1976	73	-	
Harvard (HCL)	MA, USA	1961	2002	9116	-	
Dubna (1)	Russia	1967	1996	124	-	
Moskow (ITEP)	Russia	1969	-	4162	Jul-09	
St. Petersburg	Russia	1975	-	1353	Dec-09	
Chiba	Japan	1979	2002	145	-	ocular tumors only
Tsukuba (PMRC, 1)	Japan	1983	2000	700	-	
Villigen PSI (72 MeV-Optis)	Switzerland	1984	-	5300	Dec-09	ocular tumors only
Clatterbridge	UK	1989	-	1923	Dec-09	ocular tumors only
Uppsala (2)	Sweden	1989	-	929	Dec-08	
Loma Linda (LLUMC)	CA, USA	1990	-	14000	Oct-09	
Louvain-la-Neuve	Belgium	1991	1993	21	-	ocular tumors only
Nice (CAL)	France	1991	-	3935	Dec-09	ocular tumors only
Orsay (CPO)	France	1991	-	4811	Dec-09	3936 ocular tumors
Bloomington (MPRI, 1)	IN, USA	1993	1999	34	-	ocular tumors only
iThemba LABS	South Africa	1993	-	511	Dec-09	
UCSF – CNL	CA, USA	1994	-	1200	Dec-09	ocular tumors only
Vancouver (TRIUMF)	Canada	1995	-	145	Dec-09	ocular tumors only
Villigen PSI (230 MeV)	Switzerland	1996	-	542	Dec-09	
Berlin (HMI)	Germany	1998	-	1437	Dec-09	ocular tumors only
Kashiwa (NCC)	Japan	1998	-	680	Dec-09	
Dubna (JINR, 2)	Russia	1999	-	595	Dec-09	
Boston (NPTC)	MA, USA	2001	-	4270	Oct-09	
Hyogo (HIBMC)	Japan	2001	-	2382	Nov-09	
Tsukuba (PMRC, 2)	Japan	2001	-	1586	Dec-09	
Catania (INFN-LNS)	Italy	2002	-	174	Mar-09	ocular tumors only
Tsuruga (WERC)	Japan	2002	-	56	Dec-08	
Shizuoka	Japan	2003	-	852	Dec-09	
Bloomington (MPRI, 2)	IN, USA	2004	-	890	Dec-09	
Wanjie (WPTC)	China	2004	-	977	Dec-09	
Houston (MDACC)	TX, USA	2006	-	1700	Dec-09	
Jacksonville (UFPTI)	FL, USA	2006	-	1847	Dec-09	

Continued

TABLE 1
Worldwide proton therapy facilities currently or previously in operation   (*Continued*)

Ilsan (NCC)	South Korea	2007	-	519	Dec-09
Heidelberg (HIT)	Germany	2009	-	started	Nov-09
Munich (RPTC)	Germany	2009	-	78	Dec-09
Oklahoma City (ProCurePTC)	OK, USA	2009	-	21	Dec-09
Philadelphia (UPenn)	PA, USA	2010	-	started	Jan-10

Abbreviations: CPO, Centre de Protonthérapie d'Orsay; HCL, Harvard Cyclotron Laboratory; HIT, Heidelberger Ionenstrahl-Therapiezentrum; HMI, Hahn-Meitner-Institute; INFN-LNS, Istituto Nazionale di Fisica Nucleare-Laboratori Nazionali del Sud; ITEP, Institute for Theoretical and Experimental Physics; HIBMC, Hyogo Ion Beam Medical Center; JINR, Joint Institute for Nuclear Research; LLUMC, Loma Linda University Medical Center; MDACC, MD Anderson Cancer Center; MPRI, Midwest Proton Radiotherapy Institute; NCC, National Cancer Center; NPTC, Northeast Proton Therapy Center; PMRC, Proton Medical Research Center; RPTC, Rinecker Proton Therapy Center; UFPTI, University of Florida Proton Therapy Institute; UPenn, University of Pennsylvania; WERC, Wakasa Wan Energy Research Center; WPTC, Wanjie Proton Therapy Center.

this was also where the cyclotron particle accelerator was first developed in the 1930s—a feat for which its inventor, E.O. Lawrence, was awarded the Nobel Prize. C.A. Tobias (4) initially treated the pituitary gland with proton beams that passed entirely through the head, intersecting in the target, before later on taking advantage of the Bragg peak by stopping the protons within the gland itself. In the late 1950s, the group at the Gustaf Werner Institute in Uppsala, Sweden, developed radiosurgical techniques for the treatment of brain tumors and were the first to demonstrate the use of range modulation and magnetic scanning to create a uniform region of dose capable of covering targets both longitudinally and laterally (5,6). The concepts of the rotating range modulator wheel and laterally spreading passive scattering system to achieve this same end were put into practice in 1961 at the Harvard Cyclotron Laboratory (HCL) (7). Patient-specific compensators contoured to the distal shape of the target volume were also first used here (8). All of these techniques are described in more detail in the Beam Delivery System section.

Progress was made in the ensuing decades, with many additional technologies being developed and refined. Most notable, perhaps, was the invention of the CT scanner in the 1970s, which, for the first time, enabled full, three-dimensional anatomical imaging to be performed (9,10). The development of three-dimensional treatment-planning systems at the Massachusetts General Hospital (MGH) followed shortly thereafter (11–13). However, patient treatments continued to be confined solely to facilities designed and constructed principally for high-energy physics research. As such, the proton beams tended to be fixed, and usually horizontal, in direction. The versatility provided by the isocentric gantries of conventional x-ray therapy simply wasn't available for proton beams. Only in 1990, at the Loma Linda University Medical Center (LLUMC) in California, did the first hospital-based center open its doors—an event that marked the beginning of the modern-day era of proton therapy (14).

There are now 30, mostly hospital-based, centers worldwide treating cancer patients with proton beams, in addition to eight further facilities that have done so at some time in the past. In earlier years, many were still restricted to the treatment of superficial lesions, such as those of the eye, only, owing to the limited beam energy achievable and space and cost considerations. Competition between commercial vendors has helped to overcome these issues in more recent times. In total, as many as 67,000 patients have been treated worldwide with proton therapy to date (Table 1) (15).

■ FUNDAMENTAL PHYSICS

Protons lose energy continuously in matter. Over the range of energies and in the materials of consequence for proton therapy, energy loss is principally the result of Coulombic interactions with atomic electrons; radiative losses are insignificant owing, on the atomic scale, to the proton's relatively large mass. For a proton of speed $v = \beta c$ passing through a medium of density ρ, atomic number Z, mass number A, and mean excitation energy I ($\approx 10Z$ eV), the mean rate of energy loss along the trajectory (i.e., the *stopping power*) is well described by the Bethe–Bloch equation (16):

$$
\begin{aligned}
-\left\langle \frac{dE}{dz} \right\rangle &= \frac{4\pi e^4}{m_e \beta^2 c^2} \frac{\rho Z}{A} \\
&\times \ln \left[\frac{2m_e \beta^2 c^2}{I(1-\beta^2)} - \beta^2 + a_{\text{shell}} + a_{\text{Barkas}} + a_{\text{Bloch}} \right],
\end{aligned}
\tag{1}
$$

where e and m_e are the charge and mass of the electron, respectively, and c is the speed of light in free space.

The correction a_{shell} accounts for atomic binding energies, which are otherwise neglected to a first approximation; it is smaller than 1% above proton energies of a few tens of MeV, but becomes increasingly important at lower energies (17,18). Higher-order perturbative corrections to the Born-level, leading-order term are provided by a_{Barkas} (19) and a_{Bloch} (20), which maintain 1% accuracy down to about 1 MeV. Since the electrons to which the energy is transferred have a maximum range of around 1 mm, the energy deposited by the decelerating protons can be considered to be deposited locally.

Though the theory from which Eq. 1 is derived breaks down around 1 MeV (21), it suffices to demonstrate that the origin of the Bragg peak lies in the presence of the β^2 factor in the denominator: as a proton slows down, its rate of energy loss increases in rough proportion to the inverse square of its speed. Below 1 MeV, as the proton's energy continues to fall further, its speed gradually becomes comparable to that of the outermost atomic electrons. In this realm, the stopping power decreases with further reduction in speed (22,23). Below ~1 keV, nonionizing nuclear recoil dominates the energy loss (24). Figure 3 shows the variation of stopping power and range with proton energy in water (25).

It should be emphasized that Eq. 1 is representative only of the *mean* energy loss. Fluctuations in local energy transfer conform to the highly skewed Landau–Vavilov distribution (26,27) and can be significant. Their consequence manifests as *range straggling* in proton depth–dose distributions and results in a proton range shifted to shallower depths than predicted by Eq. 1 by a few percent of that range; it is also responsible for broadening, suppression, and softening of the distal fall-off of the Bragg peak.

As can be expected, Eq. 1 demonstrates that the proton range tends to be shorter in materials of higher volumetric electron density ($\propto \rho Z/A$). However, the *mass stopping power*, $-1/\rho \langle dE/dz \rangle$, is roughly proportional to Z/A, which is a slowly decreasing function of increasing Z, though is especially large for hydrogen and especially low for the heavier elements. Thus, on a gram-for-gram basis, a proton beam generally loses more energy, and therefore deposits a higher dose, in a material of lower atomic number.

In traversing a medium, protons also suffer electromagnetic interactions with atomic nuclei. As Eq. 1 indicates, proton-stopping power is inversely proportional to the target mass (i.e., m_e). On the one hand, therefore, in comparison with electrons, the energy lost in Coulomb collisions with nuclei is negligible.

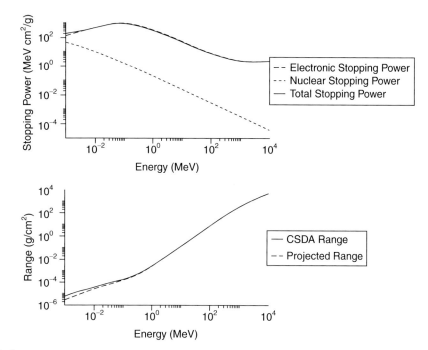

FIGURE 3

Contributions to the stopping power of protons in water from interactions with electrons and with atomic nuclei (top) and proton range in water (bottom), both plotted as a function of energy. In the latter, the range obtained by integrating the reciprocal of Eq. 1—the continuous slowing down approximation (CSDA)—is compared with the true projected range.

On the other hand, however, because of the larger target mass, the transverse scattering of protons is dominated by Coulomb interactions with nuclei. The differential cross-section at scattering angle θ is described by the Rutherford formula (28):

$$\frac{d\sigma}{d\Omega} = \frac{1}{4}\left(\frac{Ze^2}{4\pi\varepsilon_0 \, p\beta c}\right)^2 \frac{1}{\sin^4\left(\theta/2\right)}, \quad (2)$$

where p is the momentum of the incident proton. For small scattering angles the cross-section is large. The net scattering through a material is, therefore, the result of a succession of small, independent deviations. The result is that the net angle of *multiple scattering* follows a roughly Gaussian distribution, the root mean square deflection of which is (29,30):

$$\theta_{\mathrm{rms}} = \frac{13.6 \text{ MeV}}{\beta cp}\sqrt{\frac{t}{X_0}}\left(1+0.038\ln\left(\frac{t}{X_0}\right)\right), \quad (3)$$

in a layer of thickness t in the plane normal to the trajectory. Here, X_0, termed the *radiation length* of the medium, is given, to a good approximation, by (31):

$$X_0 = \frac{716A}{Z(Z+1)\ln(287/\sqrt{Z})} \text{ g cm}^{-2} \quad (4)$$

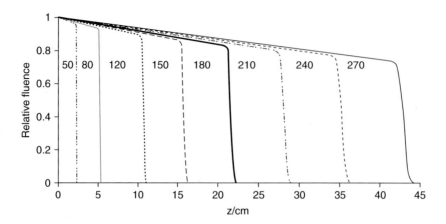

FIGURE 4
Decrease in fluence of primary protons with initial energies between 50 MeV and 270 MeV because of inelastic nuclear interactions, plotted as a function of depth in water.

The multiple-scattering distribution is, in fact, only approximately Gaussian, being modified by a long tail, roughly proportional to θ^{-3}, due to occasional single, large-angle deflections.

In addition to the elastic nuclear interactions described earlier, inelastic nuclear reactions too have a significant effect on the characteristics of proton beams. For example, approximately 21% of the energy lost in slowing down a 250-MeV proton beam in water is as a result of inelastic nuclear reactions, and about 4% for a 70-MeV beam (Figure 4) (32). These interactions produce a myriad of short-range, densely ionizing light ions, long-range protons, and a background of neutrons. The loss of primary protons from the beam tends to increase the relative dose at shallower depths.

■ **EQUIPMENT**

The elements of a proton therapy facility (Figure 5) can be divided rather broadly into three main categories: (a) the accelerator (with or without an auxiliary energy selection system) to raise the energy of the protons to the necessary level, (b) the beam transport system to convey the beam from the accelerator to the treatment room, and (c) the beam delivery system to modify the characteristics of the beam according to the particular treatment needs. Each is described, in turn, below.

Accelerator

To be viable for proton therapy, the accelerator must be capable of generating beams of sufficient energy to penetrate through tissue to the distal surface of the deepest tumors, after accounting for energy losses in the various components of the beam delivery system encountered en route. For example, a residual energy of 215 MeV at the patient surface is required for the beam to penetrate to a depth of 30 g cm^{-2}. The accelerator must, therefore, be able to produce a beam of energy between 225 MeV and 250 MeV, depending on the combination of beam-modifying elements necessary for the particular treatment. It must also be capable of supplying a beam current high enough to permit treatment times no more

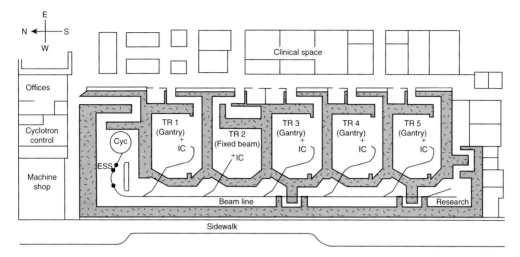

FIGURE 5
Layout of the Roberts Proton Therapy Center at the University of Pennsylvania showing the cyclotron and energy selection system (ESS), the beam transport system, and the five treatment rooms (TR 1–TR 5)—four fitted with isocentric gantries and one fitted with a fixed horizontal beam. The layout of synchrotron-based facilities is similar. (Courtesy of IBA, SA).

than a few minutes in duration. A dose rate of 2 Gy min^{-1}, for instance, demands that the beam current conveyed to the treatment be several nanoamperes. The current exiting the accelerator may need to be significantly higher, depending on the technology used and the depth and thickness of the target.

Commercial treatment systems are available that use either cyclotron or synchrotron accelerators. Both types depend on a combination of electric and magnetic fields to accelerate and bend protons around roughly circular paths. Both operate on the basis of the principle of matching the Lorentz force on the protons to the centripetal acceleration necessary for the curved trajectory, which results in the frequency, v, and radius, r, of each orbit relating to the speed, $v = \beta c$, and magnetic field strength, B, through

$$v = \frac{Be\sqrt{1 - \beta^2}}{2\pi m_\mathrm{p}},\qquad(5)$$

$$r = \frac{m_\mathrm{p}\beta c}{Be\sqrt{1 - \beta^2}},\qquad(6)$$

where m_p is the mass of the proton. The two alternatives differ, however, in the manner in which they solve these equations technically.

Other accelerator technologies, including laser-based (33) and dielectric-wall-based (34) alternatives, are also under development but have yet to be proven. They will not be discussed further here.

Cyclotron

A cyclotron accelerates charged particles by means of a high-voltage, high-frequency electric field applied between two "D"-shaped, hollow electrodes ("dees"), which are supported in a vacuum tank between the pole pieces of a large electromagnet (Figure 6). Isolated protons are produced by a centrally located, hot-filament penning ion gauge

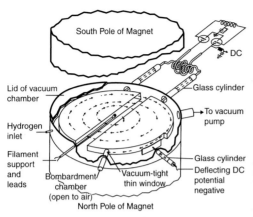 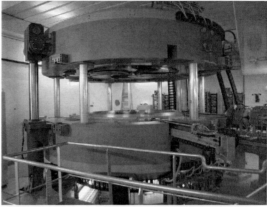

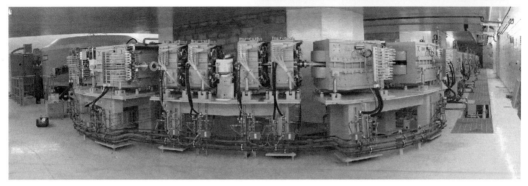

FIGURE 6
Cut-away sketch (top left) and photo (top right) showing the inner workings and components of a cyclotron, together with a photo of a cyclotron, closed for operation, and an energy selection system (bottom). (Courtesy of IBA, SA).

source and are then accelerated by the electric field into one of the dees, where the perpendicularly applied magnetic field causes them to travel on a semicircular arc. On emerging at the gap between the dees, further acceleration is provided by the alternating electric field, which is driven so as to resonate with the oscillatory frequency of the orbit (Eq. 5). Protons continue to gain energy and spiral outwards, eventually reaching a maximum energy determined by the radius of the magnetic pole pieces (Eq. 6), before being extracted.

In accelerating protons to therapeutic energies, relativistic effects become important (i.e., $\sqrt{1-\beta^2}$ deviates significantly from unity). To account for them, either the magnetic field strength must be made to increase with increasing radius in order to preserve the orbital period (as in an "isochronous" cyclotron) or the oscillatory frequency of the electric field must be made to decrease as a function of increasing radius while maintaining a constant magnetic field (as in a "synchrocyclotron") (Eq. 5). The fixed oscillatory frequency of the electric field of an isochronous cyclotron permits the generation of a continuous beam, whereas the beam from a synchrocyclotron must be pulsed, since one bunch of protons must exit before acceleration of the next

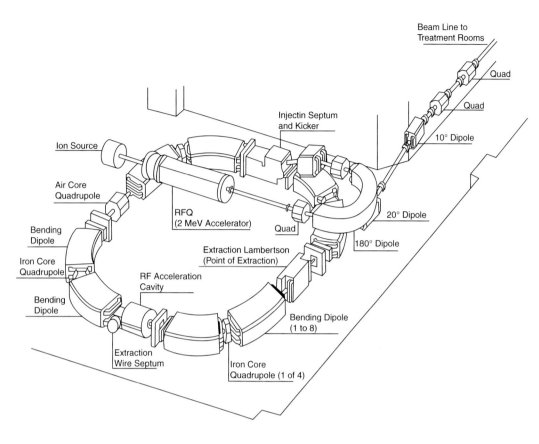

Beam Line to
Treatment Rooms

Quad

Quad

Injectin Septum
and Kicker

10° Dipole

Ion Source

20° Dipole

Air Core
Quadrupole

RFQ
(2 MeV Accelerator)   Quad

180° Dipole

Bending
Dipole

Extraction Lambertson
(Point of Extraction)

Iron Core
Quadrupole

RF Acceleration
Cavity

Bending
Dipole

Bending Dipole
(1 to 8)

Extraction
Wire Septum

Iron Core
Quadrupole (1 of 4)

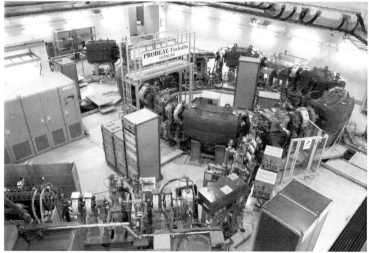

FIGURE 7

Synchrotron schematic (top) and as made by Hitachi, Ltd (bottom). (Courtesy of Hitachi, Ltd).

can begin. The former, in particular, is thus capable of producing continuous beams of high intensity, yielding a high degree of flexibility in the method of beam delivery. However, the energy at extraction is fixed, so a separate energy selector system (ESS), comprising a variable thickness degrader (typically a carbon wedge) in conjunction with magnetic energy analysis (Figure 6), is necessary to reduce the beam energy to the level desired for the given range within the patient and to control the energy spread. The secondary radiation produced in the ESS introduces additional shielding requirements.

Room-temperature isochronous cyclotrons designed for proton therapy are around 4.3 m in diameter and 200 tons in weight. By employing superconducting magnets, these parameters can be reduced to 3.1 m and 90 tons, respectively (35).

Synchrotron

A synchrotron accelerates charged particles while maintaining their trajectories along orbits of fixed radius (Figure 7). Electromagnetic resonant cavities, installed in straight sections in between dipole magnets, accelerate the particles as they circulate around the ring. The frequency of the accelerating electric field is increased as their speed increases, and this is closely coupled with the increase in the magnetic field of the dipoles (Eqs. 5 and 6). Unlike

with cyclotrons, this technique allows for the production of proton beams with a variety of energies, obviating the need for an ESS and the associated additional shielding. However, like a synchrocyclotron, a synchrotron can only deliver a pulsed beam. The intensity produced by a synchrotron is, therefore, limited. In addition, dynamic aspects of the treatment system must be designed with due respect to the duty cycle repetition rate, typically around 1 Hz. Slow extraction techniques have been developed to provide greater temporal uniformity of the beam intensity (36).

Synchrotrons are typically 1.5 to 2 times the diameter of cyclotrons of the same maximum energy.

Beam Transport System

As the accelerator accounts for a substantial portion of the equipment cost of a proton therapy center, this single resource can be best utilized if made to serve several different treatment rooms (Figure 5). This functionality is of particular value, given that the time taken to align a patient for treatment is rather longer than the treatment time itself. Thus, with multiple rooms, one patient can be undergoing treatment while others are being prepared.

The beam transport system comprises a sequence of dipole and quadrupole magnets,

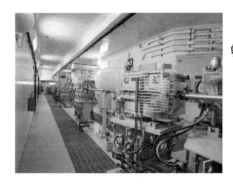 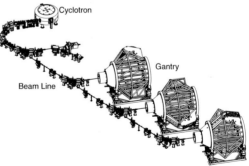

FIGURE 8
Photo (left) and schematic (right) of a beam transport system. (Courtesy of IBA, SA).

which are used to bend, steer, and focus the beam on its passage from the accelerator through an evacuated beam-pipe and on to the treatment rooms (Figure 8). Switching of the beam from one room to another is achieved by selectively energizing appropriate sets of dipole deflector magnets.

For the treatment of certain lesions, such as ocular melanomas and those requiring radiosurgery, a simple horizontal beam line is sufficient to transport the beam, once inside the room, to the patient. In the majority of cases, however, multiple beams delivered from different angles are needed to achieve the best results. In order to irradiate a patient from any desired angle, the treatment head (or "nozzle") is, therefore, affixed to an isocentric gantry, in much the same way as for conventional linac-based x-ray therapy, enabling full, 360° rotation around the treatment table (Figure 9). A further series of magnets is thus necessary to deflect the beam around the gantry and into position. Because the strength of the magnetic field dictates how small the bending radius can be (Eq. 6), this, in conjunction with the throw required to spread the beam to an adequate size laterally (Beam Delivery System section), results in a proton therapy gantry being much larger than its conventional x-ray counterpart, measuring some 10 m in diameter.

Beam Delivery System

In order to generate the desired three-dimensional dose distribution in the patient, the approximately 1-cm-wide (1σ) proton beam must next be spread and shaped laterally and range-modulated longitudinally. Two principal categories of beam delivery system exist to accomplish the former task: passive systems rely on the multiple Coulomb scattering within one or more scattering foils to broaden the beam; dynamic systems employ scanning magnets. The task of modulation in depth can be performed either by energy modulation at the accelerator (as with a synchrotron), with an ESS (as with a cyclotron), or by either of these in conjunction with range-shifting material in the nozzle.

All beam-spreading devices are housed in the gantry-mounted nozzle, together with beam-monitoring ionization chambers that detect deviations in beam position, measure the total beam current, and check the beam size and uniformity. Patient-specific beam-modifying devices (described in the following), required by all passive and some dynamic techniques, are positioned on a telescopic snout attached to the downstream end of the nozzle (Figure 9).

Passive Scattering
A passive scattering system utilizes foils of high atomic number to spread the proton beam to a diameter of up to approximately 24 cm at isocenter—adequate for covering most targets. Protons passing through a single foil of such a material will be dispersed laterally, forming an intensity distribution that is approximately Gaussian in shape. Whereas the central portion of this can be very well used for treating small targets (e.g., those in the eye) with sufficient uniformity ("single scattering"), the generation of larger field sizes, however, necessitates a "double-scattering" system.

In a double-scattering system (Figure 10), the Gaussian flux of protons from the first scatterer impinges onto a second foil located further downstream. The latter modulates this radial intensity distribution and is designed such that the combined effect of the scatterers is to create a beam of uniform lateral intensity across the patient (37). To achieve this, second scatterers are fabricated as composite devices comprising two layers: one layer of a high-Z (typically lead) and one of a low-Z material (typically polycarbonate), each of radially varying thickness. The high-Z material contributes the bulk of the scatter (Eq. 3) and is thickest at the center and roughly Gaussian in shape; the low-Z material compensates the uneven energy loss (Eq. 1) introduced as a function of radius—it is thickest at the periphery. Typically, several alternative such *contoured* second scatterers (Figure 11) are required in order to provide satisfactory lateral-dose uniformity through the entire range of possible proton energies. Proton utilization efficiency in double-scattering systems is usually close to 50%.

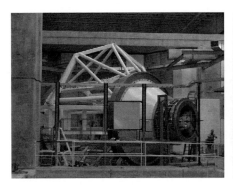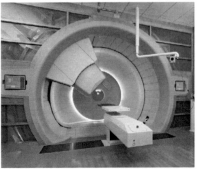

FIGURE 9
Photos showing a behind-the-scenes look of a proton therapy gantry (left) and illustrating the rotation of the gantry-mounted nozzle with telescopic snout about the table, as seen from inside a treatment room (right).

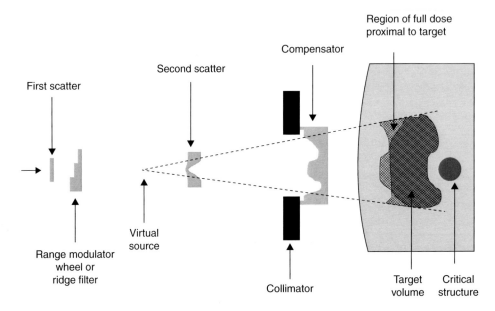

FIGURE 10
Schematic of a passive scattering system.

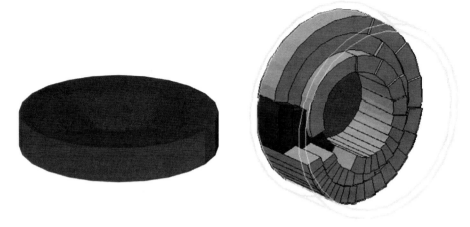

FIGURE 11

Geant4 simulation models of a contoured second scatterer (left) and a three-track range modulator wheel (right). Refs. (38, 39)

The delivery of a uniform dose throughout the range of depths of a tumor—usually much larger than the width of the Bragg peak itself—requires that modulation of the pristine Bragg peak distribution be performed. This can be accomplished by interposing absorbers of sequentially increasing thickness in the beam line and weighting the dose delivered through each such that they sum to a flat SOBP of width equal to the greatest extent in depth of the target volume (Figure 12). In practice, a range modulator wheel (7) (Figure 11) or ridge filter (40) performs this job.

A range modulator wheel comprises variable-thickness-absorber steps laid down on circular tracks that rotate through the proton beam at around 10 Hz. As for the second scatterer, a composite of a low-Z (typically polycarbonate or graphite) and a high-Z (typically lead) material is used in its fabrication. The low-Z component of each step is primarily responsible for reducing the beam energy (Eq. 1), thereby range-shifting the pristine Bragg peak to a shallower depth while keeping multiple scattering to a minimum (Eq. 3), while the high-Z component contributes primarily

to maintaining the same overall scatter from each step.

The angular width of each track step is designed to correspond closely to the weighting necessary for that pristine peak in the summation to a SOBP (Figure 12). This width thus decreases with increasing absorber thickness. In principle, a different track would need to be designed for each combination of range and modulation width. Though this is feasible, it is not always practical. Instead, some systems provide the utility to modulate the beam current from the accelerator in order to adjust the relative intensity contributed by each step within certain limits, thereby drastically reducing the number of tracks required. In the Ion Beam Applications (IBA) formulation, for example, eight tracks spread over three wheels can adequately accommodate all single- and double-scattered range–modulation combinations. Because it delivers a continuous beam, current modulation is relatively easier to control with a cyclotron.

In addition to being range-modulated, the dose distribution is also usually sculpted (typically at the 90% or 95% isodose level) to the distal

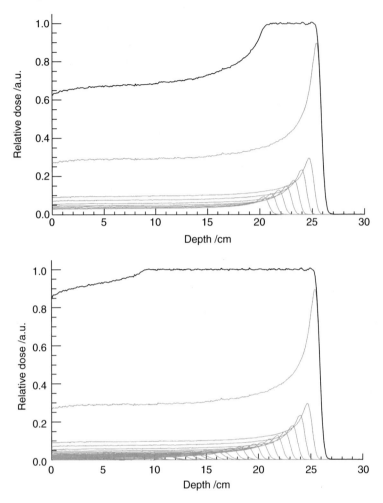

FIGURE 12
SOBP distributions for two different modulation widths and the same distal range, constructed from the component pristine peaks by terminating the beam current on different steps of the range modulator wheel track as it rotates through the beam.

surface of the target volume (Figure 10), by a portal-specific compensator (Figure 13). This comprises a block, commonly of a polymethylmethacrylate (PMMA)–type plastic, or of wax, milled out in pixels of different depth that thus provide differential range shifts transversely across the target and account for variations in the external patient shape, the internal anatomical material (Eq. 1), and the target shape itself. Commonly each pixel is *smeared* such that its depth is equal to that of the deepest in its vicinity, thereby ensuring target coverage when setup and motion uncertainties are taken into account (8).

Treatments delivered with passive systems require portal-specific collimators to shape the transverse radiation field (Figure 10). Traditionally,

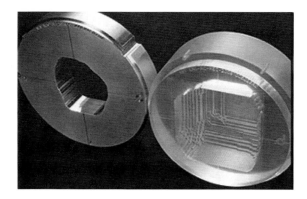

FIGURE 13
Patient portal-specific brass aperture (left) and PMMA range compensator (right). (Courtesy of .decimal®).

these have taken the form of custom-cut blocks of brass (Figure 13), based on cost, weight, and the consideration of secondary radiation production, though the use of the more versatile multileaf collimator will likely become widespread in the future. The aperture design derives from the projection of the target to isocenter plus margins that account for the size of the penumbra (typically spanning the 90– or 95–50% isodose levels) and setup uncertainties. The collimator is mounted together with the compensator on the telescopic snout, which is then translated along the beam direction in order to minimize the air gap to the surface of the patient. In this way, the broadening of the penumbra, resulting from scatter in the compensator and in the air, and on geometrical grounds, can be limited (41).

The advantage of passive scattering is the simplicity of the associated systems needed for beam monitoring and to ensure patient safety. It is also insensitive to the time structure of the beam current since the entire target is irradiated essentially simultaneously. Besides the need to manufacture patient-specific hardware, there are, however, several disadvantages. One is that by conforming the dose distribution to the distal surface of the target volume, and by delivering SOBPs of different range but the same modulation width across its transverse extent (since this is enforced by the mechanism of range modulation), a dose distribution of the same shape is necessarily imposed on the proximal surface. Normal tissues in the proximal region thus unavoidably also receive the full target dose (Figure 10), although the effect is mitigated when using multiple beams. Another is the fact that the achievable field size and the achievable range are inextricably linked: to generate a larger scattered field size, more material must be placed in the beam, but additional material in the beam reduces its maximum range. The ability to treat large, deep-seated tumors, therefore, depends on the energy reach of the accelerator. A third disadvantage is the relatively large penumbra resulting from the size of the effective source (which can be as large as 5 cm) produced by the two scatterers. The first two of these and, in some instances, the third, can be overcome through the use of a scanned beam.

Dynamic Scanning
Just as magnetic fields are used in the acceleration and transportation of the proton beam, so, too,

can they be used to deflect the beam dynamically across the target cross-section. Such dynamic systems can be implemented to deliver either "uniform" or "modulated" scanning, with the latter subclassified further into discrete spot scanning and continuous scanning techniques.

Uniform scanning

In uniform scanning (or "wobbling"), a relatively broad beam, spread by the first scatterer to around 5 cm width at isocenter, is magnetically scanned across the target volume, one depth layer at a time (42). A modulator wheel that rotates in discrete steps, rather than spinning continuously, and a series of PMMA-based binary range shifters combine to effect the transition from one layer to the next. As for double scattering, patient portal–specific collimation and range compensation are still required to define the field edge and the shape of the distal surface of the dose distribution, respectively.

The main advantage of uniform scanning compared to double scattering is that doses can be delivered both in larger field sizes (up to ~40 × 30 cm²) and at deeper depths (an additional ~1–3 g cm⁻² in range); the use of magnetic fields, rather than scattering material, to spread the beam laterally essentially decouples the achievable field size from the achievable range and avoids the range loss incurred in the scattering system. However, the principal disadvantage is that, when not limited by field size and range, the resulting dose distributions are essentially the same as achieved with double scattering, but at the expense of introducing higher sensitivity to target motion.

Modulated scanning

In discrete spot scanning, a finite pencil beam of protons is steered spot by spot to a regular array of points (often on a Cartesian lattice), with a predetermined dose being delivered to each (43) (Figure 14). To avoid nonuniformity in the dose distribution, the spot-spacing within each layer is chosen to be around 70% of the pencil beam's full width at half maximum. In between spots,

the beam is turned off. The transition between layers is performed either by changing the beam energy transported from the accelerator or by means of range shifters. If two orthogonal dipole magnets are used, adjustment of the beam energy is the time-limiting step. All spots within one layer are, therefore, delivered first, before changing the energy and repeating the process. With only one magnet, adjustments to the table position can be used to translate the beam in the third dimension (44). In this case, it is more efficient to deliver all spots along one line at multiple depths first, before changing the table position and repeating.

In continuous scanning, the beam remains on, but the current intensity or the scanning speed or both are varied as the beam sweeps across the target. The scanning is performed on a rectangular grid with a scan frequency in one direction typically 10 times higher than that in the direction perpendicular to it.

Unlike double scattering, both pencil-beam techniques present the possibility of conforming dose distributions both distally *and proximally* to targets of arbitrary shape with only a single beam (Figure 14). Objective functions can be defined to optimize scan patterns such that "single-field uniform dose" coverage is achieved. However, perhaps the defining attribute of pencil-beam scanning is that it permits the delivery of "intensity-modulated proton therapy" (IMPT)—the proton equivalent of IMRT. With IMPT, the scan patterns for all beams in a plan are optimized simultaneously, often with respect to additional dose constraints on organs at risk (OARs), such that their combination delivers the desired dose distributions to both the target volume and the OARs (45). The dose distribution in the target can thus be designed either to be uniform (though the contribution from each beam may be highly inhomogeneous) or to incorporate a simultaneously boost. Moreover, IMPT realizes the full potential of proton beams to provide highly localized dose distributions because it encompasses not only intensity modulation, as with IMRT, but

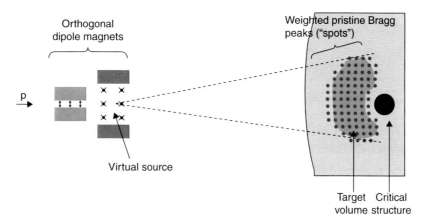

FIGURE 14
Schematic of a dynamic scanning system.

also energy modulation, which vastly increases its dose-shaping ability (46).

Additional benefits of pencil-beam scanning include the absence of scatterers and apertures from the beam line, which removes the secondary radiation contribution that is otherwise generated by nuclear reactions within these devices, and the absence of compensators, as well as apertures, which saves both time and resources. However, generating very narrow pencil beams that result in an optimal lateral dose fall-off is technically challenging. Furthermore, the increased complexity of the treatment delivery renders the effect of organ motion an important concern in planning treatment (47,48).

Motion errors are currently addressed by two primary means: beam gating and repainting. With gating, the beam is turned off when the target has moved out of the bounds for which the treatment plan has been calculated and turns on again when it returns (49). By repainting, either single spots, individual layers, or the entire treatment volume are scanned multiple times over. Although both approaches reduce errors introduced by target motion, both can also result in

the therapeutic dose taking a significantly longer time to deliver compared to passive scattering techniques. However, much present-day research and development work is being invested in this area, so practical solutions will, in all likelihood, be forthcoming (50,51).

■ TREATMENT PLANNING

As for conventional x-ray treatments, the planning process for proton therapy begins with a planning CT scan of the patient immobilized in the treatment position, followed by delineation of target volumes and OARs in the computerized planning system. Additional positron emission tomography (PET) and/or MRI studies may facilitate this. However, the planning strategies from there on need not be the same, because the beam characteristics and delivery methods for protons differ markedly from those for x-rays, as discussed in the Fundamental Physics and Equipment sections. Several considerations pertinent to proton therapy treatment planning are described below.

Nevertheless, this additional degree of freedom is often available to the planner in choosing how best to direct the beams. In addition, x-ray-based treatment planning is restricted by the common need to use paired, often near-opposing, beam directions to achieve dose homogeneity. This is not necessary in proton planning. Non-coplanar beam arrangements, such as the inclusion of vertex beams, can, therefore, be used a greater effect.

■ FUTURE DIRECTIONS

Though many of the aspects of proton therapy described previously are now relatively mature, there is undoubtedly much scope for future innovation. Two areas of development that have shown much promise, have attracted considerable interest and have not already been alluded to in the preceding text are proton radiography and PET. The potential role of each is, therefore, discussed in the following.

Proton Radiography

In order to perform routine proton imaging, beams of energies higher than are currently available clinically, and sufficient to penetrate the largest patient, must be generated. Assuming this will likely be possible in the future, two purposes may then be served. First, detection of protons transmitted through the patient in the treatment position can be used to facilitate localization (58,59). At present, a retractable x-ray tube mounted in the nozzle coaxially with the proton beam is often used to verify the alignment of the beam relative to the patient prior to treatment. Any displacement between the x-ray- and proton-beam axes thus introduces systematic errors. By contrast, direct use of the proton beam would enable images to be acquired with exactly the same geometrical conditions as encountered during treatment. Second, proton CT could be used to measure proton-stopping powers directly for voxelized patient anatomies (60). This would

eliminate the need to construct inexact calibration curves and the associated uncertainties (Heterogeneities section) (61).

For both modes of utilization, multiple scattering and range straggling (Fundamental Physics section) in the patient tend to limit, respectively, the achievable spatial and density resolution. However, techniques to reconstruct the most likely path (62,63), and to measure the residual range, of each proton passing through the patient have been demonstrated to yield considerable improvements in both, resulting in spatial resolution that is comparable to that achievable with x-rays and density resolution that is largely superior (64,65). Possible designs for proton CT scanners have already been conceived (66), though have yet to be realized commercially.

Positron Emission Tomography

During treatment, the nuclear interactions of protons with tissue result in the production of small amounts of radioisotopes, including ^{11}C ($T_{1/2}$ ~20 minutes), ^{13}N ($T_{1/2}$ ~10 minutes), and ^{15}O ($T_{1/2}$ ~2 minutes), along the path of the beam. PET can be used to detect the gamma rays produced by the annihilation with atomic electrons of the positrons produced in their subsequent nuclear decays (67,68). Although the distribution of measured PET activity does not translate directly into the distribution of dose—and, indeed, the existence of an energy threshold implies there is actually no activation near the end of the proton range—the accuracy of the treatment delivered can nevertheless be monitored by comparing this measured activity distribution with that calculated by a treatment-planning system or by Monte Carlo simulation. By this mechanism, it is possible both to assess range uncertainties in the treatment-planning calculations and to track, noninvasively, changes to the anatomy of the patient or to the tumor that, if sufficiently large, may warrant the acquisition of a further planning CT scan. The shortness of the half-lives of the radioisotopes produced, however, dictates that such PET imaging must take place either during or immediately after treatment—and ideally, therefore, in the treatment room itself. Investigations into such practicalities are ongoing (69,70).

CONCLUSIONS

Proton beams possess fundamental physical characteristics that place them at a distinct radiotherapeutic advantage when compared to conventional x-rays. Unlike x-ray beams, for which optimization of the fluence can only be carried out in the two transverse dimensions, proton-beam fluence can also be regulated in depth. Because of the capacity for full, three-dimensional fluence modulation within each beam, proton therapy permits an increased dose to be delivered to a target volume for given doses to neighboring sensitive structures, and therefore promises improved local control and disease-free survival. For a given target dose, it also results in lower doses being delivered to normal tissues and, thus, has the potential to reduce morbidity, increase tolerance when used in conjunction with chemotherapy, and improve quality of life. Though being of special importance for pediatric patients, these far-reaching consequences are, of course, to the great benefit of all.

Various, well-established delivery systems exist that exploit the characteristic features of proton beams. As with other forms of radiation therapy, though, the principal challenge of the technology is in ensuring that calculated treatment plans are accurately reflected in the dose distributions delivered to patients. This is of particular concern for proton therapy because of the precise nature of the treatment. Nonetheless, the associated issues are well known, and refinements to delivery techniques and advancements with treatment-planning and quality-assurance systems are being made all the time to address them. As the accuracy and robustness of proton therapy continue to improve, so the day when its immense power will be harnessed to the full draws ever nearer.

REFERENCES

1. Miralbell R, Lomax A, Cella L, Schneider U. Potential reduction of the incidence of radiation-induced second cancers by using proton beams in the treatment of pediatric tumors. *Int J Radiat Oncol Biol Phys.* 2002;54(3):824–829.
2. Kirsch DG, Tarbell NJ. Conformal radiation therapy for childhood CNS tumors. *Oncologist.* 2004; 9(4):442–450.
3. Wilson RR. Radiological use of fast protons. *Radiology.* 1946;47(5):487–491.
4. Tobias CA, Lawrence JH, Born JL, et al. Pituitary irradiation with high-energy proton beams. *Cancer Res.* 1958;18:121–134.
5. Larsson B, Leksell L, Rexed B, Sourander P, Mair W, Andersson B. The high-energy proton beam as a neurosurgical tool. *Nature.* 1958;182(4644):1222–1223.
6. Larsson B. Radiological properties of beams of high-energy protons. *Radiat Res Suppl.* 1967;7:304–311.
7. Koehler AM, Schneider RJ, Sisterson JM. Range modulators for protons and heavy ions. *Nucl Instrum Methods.* 1975;131:437–440.
8. Wagner MS. Automated range compensation for proton therapy. *Med Phys.* 1982;9(5):749–752.
9. Hounsfield GN. Computerized transverse axial scanning (tomography). 1. Description of system. *Br J Radiol.* 1973;46(552):1016–1022.
10. Ambrose J. Computerized transverse axial scanning (tomography). 2. Clinical application. *Br J Radiol.* 1973;46(552):1023–1047.
11. Goitein M, Abrams M. Multi-dimensional treatment planning: I. Delineation of anatomy. *Int J Radiat Oncol Biol Phys.* 1983;9(6):777–787.
12. Goitein M, Abrams M, Rowell D, Pollari H, Wiles J. Multi-dimensional treatment planning: II. Beam's eye-view, back projection, and projection through CT sections. *Int J Radiat Oncol Biol Phys.* 1983; 9(6):789–797.
13. Goitein M, Miller T. Planning proton therapy of the eye. *Med Phys.* 1983;10(3):275–283.
14. Slater JM, Archambeau JO, Miller DW, Notarus MI, Preston W, Slater JD. The proton treatment center at Loma Linda University Medical Center: rationale for and description of its development. *Int J Radiat Oncol Biol Phys.* 1992;22(2):383–389.

15. Particle Therapy Co Operative Group. PTCOG Web site. http://ptcog.web.psi.ch/ptcentres.html. Accessed in May 2010.

16. Bethe HA. Zur Theorie des Durchgangs schneller Korpuskularstrahlen durch Materie. *Ann Phys.* 1930; 397:325–400.

17. Bichsel H. Stopping power and ranges of fast ions in heavy elements. *Phys Rev, A.* 1992;46(9):5761–5773.

18. Barkas WH, Berger MJ. *Tables of energy losses and ranges of heavy charged particles.* Washington, DC: National Academy of Sciences—National Research Council; 1964. Report NASA-SP-3013.

19. Barkas WH, Birnbaum W, Smith FM. Mass-ratio method applied to the measurement of *L*-meson masses and the energy balance in pion decay. *Phys Rev.* 1956;101:778–795.

20. International Commission on Radiation Units & Measurements. *Stopping power and ranges for protons and alpha particles.* Bethesda, MD: ICRU; 1993. ICRU Report No. 49.

21. Anderson HH, Ziegler JF. Hydrogen: stopping powers and ranges in all elements. In: *Stopping powers and ranges of Ions in Matter. Vol. 3.* New York: Pergamon Press; 1977.

22. Lindhard J. Kgl. *Danske Videnskab. Selskab. Mat. Fys Medd.* 1954;28, No. 8.

23. Lindhard J, Scharff M, Schiøtt HE. *Danske Videnskab. Selskab, Mat.-Fys. Medd.* 1963;33, No. 14.

24. Ziegler JF, Biersac JF, Littmark U. In: *The stopping and range of Ions in Solids.* New York: Pergamon Press; 1985.

25. Berger MJ. [NIST]. Stopping-power and range tables for electrons, protons, and helium ions. Available at http://www.nist.gov/physlab/data/radiation.cfm. Accessed in May 2010.

26. Landau LD. On the energy loss of fast particles by ionization. *J Exp Phys. (USSR).* 1944;8:201–205.

27. Vavilov PV. Ionization losses of high-energy heavy particles. *Sov Phys. JETP.* 1957;5:749–751.

28. Rutherford E. The scattering of α and β particles by matter and the structure of the atom. *Philosophical Magazine.* 1911;Series 6, vol. 21:669–688.

29. Highland VL. Some practical remarks on multiple scattering. *Nucl Instrum Methods.* 1975;129:497–499. Erratum. *Nucl Instrum Methods.* 1979;161:171–171.

30. Lynch GR, Dahl OI. Approximations to multiple Coulomb scattering. *Nucl Instrum Methods.* 1991;B58:6–10.

31. Amsler C, Particle Data Group. Review of particle physics. *Phys Lett.* 2008;B667:267–280.

32. Ulmer W. Theoretical aspects of energy–range relations, stopping power and energy straggling of protons. *Radiat Phys and Chem.* 2007;76:1089–1107.

33. Ma CM, Veltchev I, Fourkal E, et al. Development of a laser-driven accelerator for cancer therapy. *Laser Phys.* 2006;16:1–8.

34. Caporaso GJ, Mackie TR, Sampayan S, et al. A compact linac for intensity modulated proton therapy based on a dielectric wall accelerator. *Phys Med.* 2008; 24(2):98–101.

35. Klein H, Baumgarten C, Geisler A, et al. New superconducting cyclotron driven scanning proton therapy systems. *Nucl Instrum Methods Phys Res.* 2005;B 241:721–726.

36. Hiramoto K, Nishi M. Resonant beam extraction scheme with constant separatrix. *Nucl Instrum Methods Phys Res.* 1992;A 322:154–160.

37. Koehler AM, Schneider RJ, Sisterson JM. Flattening of proton dose distributions for large-field radiotherapy. *Med Phys.* 1977;4(4):297–301.

38. Agostinelli S, Allison J, Amako K, et al.; Geant4 Collaboration. Geant4—a simulation toolkit. *Nucl Instrum Methods Phys Res.* 2003;A 506:250–303.

39. Allison J, Amako K, Apostolakis J, et al.; Geant4 Collaboration. Geant4 developments and applications. *IEEE Trans Nucl Sci.* 2006;53:270–278.

40. Chu WT, Ludewigt BA, Renner TR. Instrumentation for treatment of cancer using proton and light-ion beams. *Rev Sci Instrum.* 1993;64:2055–2122.

41. Sisterson JM, Urie MM, Koehler AM, Goitein M. Distal penetration of proton beams: the effects of air gaps between compensating bolus and patient. *Phys Med Biol.* 1989;34(9):1309–1315.

42. Chu W, McEvoy M, Nyman M, et al. Wobbler dosimetry for the biomedical program at the LBL Bevalac. *IEEE Trans Nucl Sci.* 1985;NS-32:3324–3326.

43. Kanai T, Kawachi K, Kumamoto Y, et al. Spot scanning system for proton radiotherapy. *Med Phys.* 1980; 7(4):365–369.

44. Pedroni E, Bacher R, Blattmann H, et al. The 200-MeV proton therapy project at the Paul Scherrer Institute: conceptual design and practical realization. *Med Phys.* 1995;22(1):37–53.

45. Oelfke U, Bortfeld T. Inverse planning for photon and proton beams. *Med Dosim.* 2001;26(2):113–124.

46. Lomax A. Intensity modulation methods for proton radiotherapy. *Phys Med Biol.* 1999;44(1):185–205.

47. Phillips MH, Pedroni E, Blattmann H, Boehringer T, Coray A, Scheib S. Effects of respiratory motion on dose uniformity with a charged particle scanning method. *Phys Med Biol.* 1992;37(1):223–234.

48. Bortfeld T, Jokivarsi K, Goitein M, Kung J, Jiang SB. Effects of intra-fraction motion on IMRT dose delivery: statistical analysis and simulation. *Phys Med Biol.* 2002;47(13):2203–2220.

49. Lu HM, Brett R, Sharp G, et al. A respiratory-gated treatment system for proton therapy. *Med Phys.* 2007;34(8):3273–3278.

50. Furukawa T, Inaniwa T, Sato S, et al. Design study of a raster scanning system for moving target irradiation in heavy-ion radiotherapy. *Med Phys.* 2007;34(3):1085–1097.

51. Bert C, Saito N, Schmidt A, Chaudhri N, Schardt D, Rietzel E. Target motion tracking with a scanned particle beam. *Med Phys.* 2007;34(12):4768–4771.

52. Hong L, Goitein M, Bucciolini M, et al. A pencil beam algorithm for proton dose calculations. *Phys Med Biol.* 1996;41(8):1305–1330.

53. Pedroni E, Scheib S, Böhringer T, et al. Experimental characterization and physical modelling of the dose distribution of scanned proton pencil beams. *Phys Med Biol.* 2005;50(3):541–561.

54. Paganetti H, Jiang H, Parodi K, Slopsema R, Engelsman M. Clinical implementation of full Monte Carlo dose calculation in proton beam therapy. *Phys Med Biol.* 2008;53(17):4825–4853.

55. Tourovsky A, Lomax AJ, Schneider U, Pedroni E. Monte Carlo dose calculations for spot scanned proton therapy. *Phys Med Biol.* 2005;50(5):971–981.

56. Schneider U, Pedroni E, Lomax A. The calibration of CT Hounsfield units for radiotherapy treatment planning. *Phys Med Biol.* 1996;41(1):111–124.

57. Schaffner B, Pedroni E. The precision of proton range calculations in proton radiotherapy treatment planning: experimental verification of the relation between CT-HU and proton stopping power. *Phys Med Biol.* 1998;43(6):1579–1592.

58. Schneider U, Pedroni E. Proton radiography as a tool for quality control in proton therapy. *Med Phys.* 1995;22(4):353–363.

59. Schneider U, Besserer J, Pemler P, et al. First proton radiography of an animal patient. *Med Phys.* 2004;31(5):1046–1051.

60. Zygmanski P, Gall KP, Rabin MS, Rosenthal SJ. The measurement of proton stopping power using proton-cone-beam computed tomography. *Phys Med Biol.* 2000;45(2):511–528.

61. Schneider U, Pemler P, Besserer J, Pedroni E, Lomax A, Kaser-Hotz B. Patient specific optimization of the relation between CT-hounsfield units and proton stopping power with proton radiography. *Med Phys.* 2005;32(1):195–199.

62. Schneider U, Pedroni E. Multiple Coulomb scattering and spatial resolution in proton radiography. *Med Phys.* 1994;21(11):1657–1663.

63. Williams DC. The most likely path of an energetic charged particle through a uniform medium. *Phys Med Biol.* 2004;49(13):2899–2911.

64. Schulte RW, Bashkirov V, Klock MC, et al. Density resolution of proton computed tomography. *Med Phys.* 2005;32(4):1035–1046.

65. Talamonti C, Reggioli V, Bruzzi M, et al. Proton radiography for clinical applications. *Nucl Instrum Methods Phys Res.* 2010;A 612:571–575.

66. Schulte R, Bashkirov V, Tianfang L, et al. Conceptual design of a proton computed tomography system for applications in proton radiation therapy. *IEEE Trans Nucl Sci.* 2004;51:866–872.

67. Hishikawa Y, Kagawa K, Murakami M, Sakai H, Akagi T, Abe M. Usefulness of positron-emission tomographic images after proton therapy. *Int J Radiat Oncol Biol Phys.* 2002;53(5):1388–1391.

68. Enghardt W, Crespo P, Fiedler F, et al. Charged hadron tumour therapy monitoring by means of PET. *Nucl Instrum Methods Phys Res.* 2004;A 525:284–288.

69. Parodi K, Paganetti H, Shih HA, et al. Patient study of *in vivo* verification of beam delivery and range, using positron emission tomography and computed tomography imaging after proton therapy. *Int J Radiat Oncol Biol Phys.* 2007;68(3):920–934.

70. Parodi K, Bortfeld T, Haberer T. Comparison between in-beam and offline positron emission tomography imaging of proton and carbon ion therapeutic irradiation at synchrotron- and cyclotron-based facilities. *Int J Radiat Oncol Biol Phys.* 2008;71(3):945–956.

demos
MEDICAL

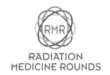

RADIATION
MEDICINE ROUNDS

Biology of Proton Therapy: Old and New Considerations

Michael J. Eblan and Keith A. Cengel*

University of Pennsylvania, Philadelphia, PA

■ ABSTRACT

The physical characteristics of photon radiation dose distributions make it difficult to achieve a tumoricidal radiation dose without unacceptably damaging the surrounding normal tissues. Proton radiotherapy allows a greater degree of spatial control over radiation dose distribution, permitting the delivery of increasing doses of ionizing radiation to malignant tumors while sparing dose to critical normal tissues. Clinical use of proton radiotherapy for cancer patients has operated under the assumption that the relative biological effectiveness (RBE, the ratio of cell death from proton/photon radiotherapy) for protons is close to unity to conventional photon radiotherapy. Patient outcomes using this assumption have been quite favorable. Nevertheless, preclinical data indicate that protons can have RBE values as high as 2 to 3, especially when protons are delivered with lower fraction sizes (2–3 Gy) and at depths near the end of a proton's track. In addition, there are likely cell- and tissue-specific interactions of protons that produce a unique gene activation profile as compared with photons, creating cell and tissue context-dependent influences on proton radiobiology. Finally, there are very limited data on the impact of proton-specific interactions in combined modality chemoradiotherapy using either cytotoxic or molecularly targeted agents. As a larger number of patients with diverse tumor types and locations are treated with protons, in an age where multimodality, molecularly targeted therapies are now standard of care for most definitive cancer treatments, it is essential to more clearly delineate the cell and tissue contexts that lead to high proton RBE values and determine the clinical applicability of these phenomena.

Keywords: proton radiobiology, relative biological effectiveness, combined modality therapy

*Corresponding author, Department of Radiation Oncology, University of Pennsylvania, 180G John Morgan Building, 3620 Hamilton Walk, Philadelphia, PA 19104

E-mail address: Keith.Cengel@uphs.upenn.edu

Radiation Medicine Rounds 1:3 (2010) 441–454.
DOI: 10.5003/2151–4208.1.3.441

demosmedpub.com/rmr

■ INTRODCUTION

Over the past 114 years, the majority of preclinical radiobiological studies and clinical radiotherapy treatments have been performed using either photons (x-rays or gamma rays) or electrons to deliver the radiation dose. Unfortunately, the physical limitations on the distribution of radiation dose imposed by photon and/or electron beam therapy make it difficult to achieve a tumoricidal radiation dose without unacceptably damaging the surrounding normal tissues. The main attraction of radiation therapy with charged particles such as protons is that the physical characteristics of these particles allow a much greater degree of spatial control over radiation dose distribution. Because the majority of the proton radiation dose occurs with a low ionization density, except near the end of the proton track length (the Bragg Peak region, Figure 1), it has been hypothesized that protons are radiobiologically similar to both photons and electrons in terms of normal tissue and tumor tissue radiation dose-response characteristics. Thus, in theory, we should be able to apply radiation therapy experience from the past century quite readily to adapt proton beams to the therapy of cancer patients.

Clinical use of proton radiotherapy for cancer patients has operated with the assumption that the relative biological effectiveness (RBE, the ratio for a particular biological effect from proton/photon radiotherapy) for protons is close to unity (1–4). Patient outcomes using this assumption have, thus far, been quite favorable. However, many of these treatments have been performed using a combination of photon and proton radiotherapy. In addition, the vast majority of these treatments were performed with passively scattered proton beams delivered to a limited number of body sites. As increasing numbers of patients with diverse cancer types and anatomical tumor locations are treated with newer proton technologies, such as tumor treatment with thin beams of energy-modulated protons (e.g., "pencil beam" scanning), more studies are needed to confirm if the assumption about proton RBE continues to be clinically applicable.

■ RBE AS A MEASURE OF PROTON EFFECTS

RBE is defined as the dose of a reference radiation that produces a particular effect or outcome divided by the dose of the investigated radiation for this same effect. In the modern era, the reference radiation is ^{60}Co due to its widespread availability, radiobiological similarity to MV photons produced by a linear accelerator and the constancy of this form of radiation. Also, ^{60}Co gamma rays are a stable form of radiation that is the same in all places and at all times. Because of the emerging use of proton radiotherapy in human patients, previous in vitro and in vivo studies have attempted to define the RBE for protons using cell culture and animal models (reviewed in (1–4)).

In general, the in vitro studies show significantly more variability in RBE than the in vivo studies. Many of these studies inadequately detail or do not describe the quality assurance steps taken to verify the accuracy and dosimetry of the proton irradiation setup. Overall, the in vitro studies suggest an RBE value of 1.1 to 1.4 and the in vivo studies suggest an RBE value of 1.0 to 1.2. One potential explanation for the range of RBE values obtained using in vitro models is variation

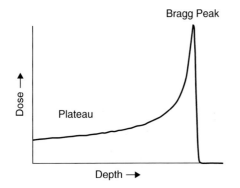

FIGURE 1
Depth dose distribution for monoenergetic protons.

resulting from the differences in specific cell handling and irradiation conditions between the photon irradiation sources (often fixed vertical beam) and proton irradiation sources (often fixed horizontal beam). Another explanation may be the difference in the measured endpoints. For in vitro studies, the endpoint is often loss of clonogenic potential in individual cells. The in vivo endpoints involve measuring tissue response, which may have a different degree of inherent variability in measurement. Nevertheless, clinical proton doses are commonly prescribed using RBE as a single, scalar multiplier to create a cobalt gray equivalent (CGE) dose.

There are significant drawbacks to using a single, scalar multiplier to convert a proton dose to a CGE dose. Conceptually, RBE is fairly robust when a single binary effect is considered, such as cell survival or cell death. However, it deteriorates as the RBE concept is applied to multifaceted, graded effects. Thus, the major strength of RBE used in this way is also its greatest weakness. A single RBE value is used to convert a proton to a photon dose equivalent that can be used for radiation protection calculations and for estimating the potential effects of a particular dose of proton radiation. However, using a single scalar multiplier for all proton radiation doses to all cell and tissue types ignores potentially important biological effects that may not be subtle. These effects could clinically manifest as either increased toxicity or decreased tumor cure rate. If a more complex model of RBE was incorporated into treatment planning, proton treatments could be delivered in a way that maximally exploits radiobiologic differences of protons as compared with photons, leading to an increase in the therapeutic index of proton radiation. However, it remains unclear that any benefit of such modeling would be large enough to merit the increased complexity of treatment planning and delivery.

■ PHYSICAL CONTRIBUTIONS TO PROTON RADIOBIOLOGY

The potential radiobiological differences between protons and photons can be considered in two conceptually separated areas. The first involves the physical differences in the track structure of deposited dose and secondary particle distributions between proton and photon beams. The second area involves differences in the impact of these physical proton beam properties on specific cells and tissues as determined by tissue- and cell-specific differences in radiobiologic response characteristics, which will be discussed in the next section. The primary proton particles deposit dose through ionization and excitation of atomic electrons and through interactions with nuclei, both radiative (bremsstrahlung) and collisional. The nuclear interactions can result in the production of secondary heavier charged particles such as alpha particles or neutrons. These secondary particles are generated primarily in the entrance dose (plateau) portion of the proton dose distribution and can have a much higher RBE than the primary protons. In the Bragg peak region, the proton dose is deposited through scattered electrons and from the protons themselves. Thus, the physical characteristics of the RBE of the proton beam may vary in different regions of the proton dose distribution due to differences in the RBE of the scattered particles. In addition, as the protons slow down, the probability of interacting with electrons increases, creating the Bragg peak portion of the proton dose distribution (Figure 1). Within the Bragg peak, the linear energy transfer (LET) of protons increases significantly, giving rise to another potential area of higher RBE.

RBE and LET Versus Depth in Spread Out Bragg Peak

In general, RBE increases as LET increases for ionizing radiation, up to a maximal limit of 100 keV/μm. For proton beams, the absorbed dose for higher energy protons (>100 MeV) that contributes to the majority of the dose used in proton radiotherapy is deposited with LETs in the range of 0.1 to 1 keV/μm (Figure 2). This LET spectrum is highly similar to the LET spectrum of electrons

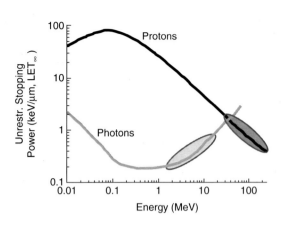

FIGURE 2

LET for photons versus protons. LET values are obtained using PSTAR (http://physics.nist.gov/Phys RefData/Star/Text/PSTAR.html) and ESTAR (http://physics.nist.gov/PhysRefData/Star/Text/ESTAR.html) for protons and Compton-scattered electrons, respectively. The shaded areas represent commonly used treatment energies for comparison.

that are produced from Compton-scattering by ^{60}Co photons. For protons with energies less than 100 MeV, the LET increases to a maximal value approaching 100 keV/μm for protons in the terminal Bragg peak portion of the depth dose distribution. Thus, lower incident/maximal proton energies lead to more superficial Bragg peaks and a relatively higher percentage of the total radiation dose delivered with a higher LET. Indeed, experiments with monoenergetic protons confirm that the increased LET can lead to RBE values as high as 2 to 3.

Most of the clinical proton treatments performed to date have used range modulation techniques to create a spread out Bragg peak (SOBP).

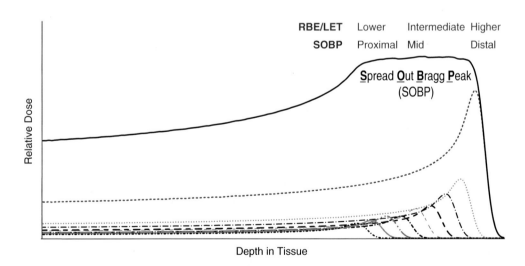

FIGURE 3

Spread out Bragg Peak. The polyenergetic SOBP is made up of multiple, smaller monoenergetic Bragg peaks. This creates an SLE spectrum where the terminal SOBP has a higher average LET than the proximal SOBP. (Geant4 simulation data for SOBP is courtesy of J. McDonough.)

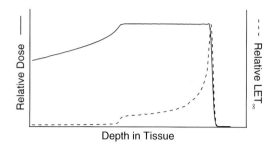

FIGURE 4

LET versus dose for SOBP. (Geant4 simulation data for SOBP/LET is courtesy of E.S. Diffenderfer.)

The SOBP is essentially a summation of multiple individual Bragg peaks with the dominant (highest fluence) peak as the highest energy and multiple smaller (less fluence) Bragg peaks filling in the dose at more superficial depths (Figure 3). Within the SOBP, the average LET slowly increases as the proportion of energy deposited from Bragg peak versus plateau protons increases until the final few millimeters, where the LET rises sharply (Figure 4). Preclinical studies have used the plateau or mid-spread-out Bragg peak portions of the depth-dose distribution to create a relatively homogenous radiation dose for a specific cell or tissue. These studies suggest that the difference in LET between plateau and mid-SOBP protons leads to an increased RBE of approximately 10%. The average LET also varies with the overall depth and width of the SOBP, with more superficial, narrower (less range modulation) SOBP having a higher average LET spectrum. Again, experimental data to date confirm that the RBE values for both in vitro and in vivo endpoints follow the same trend as the LET. For both types of endpoints, RBE increases throughout the course of an SOBP and is slightly higher in the SOBP than the plateau portions of the proton dose distribution, with values up to 1.4 to 1.6 in the distal SOBP (5–7).

Finally, there are limited data indicating that high RBE values may be obtained when using the higher energy, entrance dose (plateau) portion of the proton beam for beam energies of 1 GeV. The clinical significance of these findings is uncertain (AR Kennedy, personal communication). Most studies with protons have used a limited number of beam energies and SOBPs with a single cell line or endpoint, making it difficult to determine the overall accuracy of using LET and physical beam properties to predict RBE for treatment planning purposes. Indeed, there are several lines of evidence suggesting LET alone may be insufficient to predict cell survival. For example, in vitro experiments with V79 cells demonstrate that protons and helium ions of equal LET can give different survival levels (8).

The approximation that most of the energy deposited by therapeutic protons is with lower LETs that are consistent with previous photon radiation experience is most valid for deeper tumors treated with higher energy proton beams. In clinical treatment of head and neck cancers and other superficial tumors, most of the treatment volume is relatively superficial (e.g., 1–4 cm) and the energy spectrum of the protons used will be less than 70 MeV. The lower overall energy spectrum combines with the increased sharpness of the Bragg peaks/ lesser LET-averaging effects of straggling to make the average LET of these superficial SOBP higher than the average LET for SOBP used in treating tumor volumes at depths of 20 to 25 cm, as would be used for a typical prostate cancer proton treatment. One correction method uses a weighting function of LET for different proton energies to create a RBE weighting function (9). Treatment plans for hypopharynx cancer created using a LET-corrected RBE dose weighting algorithm show significantly higher biological doses for the same given proton dose as compared with plans created using a single, scalar RBE multiplier (10). However, models that use only LET and/or other beam characteristics to create a variable RBE function do not include potentially critical information on cell or tissue-specific factors that may determine the biological impact of proton radiation.

■ CELL- AND TISSUE-SPECIFIC CONTRIBUTIONS TO PROTON RBE

The second area of concern over proton RBE is biological. There is increasing evidence of tissue and cancer-cell type-specific differences in proton radiobiology. One critically important aspect in the radiocurability for tumors is therapeutic index, which is the ratio of damage to malignant versus normal tissues. Protons can increase the therapeutic index of radiotherapy due to the lack of exit dose and other physical properties of the proton beam, providing protons with spatial advantages over photons. Thus, the increased spatial advantages of protons allow the delivery of higher tumor doses for the same dose to the surrounding normal tissues. Another potential and less explored advantage of protons is in using the higher LET of protons to maximize biological response to treatment. For protons, many of the preclinical studies using in vitro methods have used Chinese Hamster (V79) cells. Therefore, data is lacking examining the factors that contribute to proton radiosensitivity in normal or malignant human cell lines. A limited number of studies have shown that the higher LET protons may provide a benefit for less photon radiosensitive cancers. However, this benefit is less than that observed using carbon ions, where particle radiations with a higher proportion of the total energy are deposited as higher LET.

In general, as the LET increases, there is larger increase in radiosensitivity for cells with a high DNA repair capacity that are less photon radiosensitive than for cells with a low DNA repair capacity or low proliferation rate that are more photon radiosensitive (11–13). Cancer cells that are less radiosensitive often have a high DNA repair capacity (14). There is evidence from in vitro studies in rodent and human cancer cell lines that the differences in radiosensitivity using photons is not as significant for particle radiation with increased LET. Early experiments using highly radiosensitive fibroblasts from a patient with Ataxia Telangiectasia found that neon or argon ions with LET up to 100 to 200 keV/μm showed a smaller increase in RBE as compared to the increase in RBE seen with high LET radiation in a less radiosensitive human fibroblast cell line (15). With high LET charged particles such as helium ions, investigators have found a higher RBE for human cancer cells that are less photon radiosensitive as measured by in vitro survival assays for glioma, prostate, and colon cancer cells (5,16). Other investigators have found that as LET increases from 20 to 100 keV/μm, the RBE of carbon ions increases in a variety of human cancer cells, including glioblastoma, lung, cervical, and esophageal squamous cell carcinomas and lung, ovarian, and endometrial adenocarcinomas (12,17,18).

For 6 to 30 keV/μm protons, a similar trend has been found using human head and neck squamous cell carcinoma, melanoma, and glioblastoma cell lines (17,19,20). Interestingly, studies of normal tissues have found less of a difference in RBE, although this may be reflective of the trend of in vivo studies to show less proton RBE variability (6,7,21,22). Thus, increased LET can lead to increased sensitivity of cancer cells that are more resistant to photon radiation. This increased radiation sensitivity may improve the therapeutic index of charged particle radiation over and above what could be expected given the spatial advantages of increased dose to tumor compared with normal tissue. Because the overall or average LET of proton radiotherapy treatments is less than carbon ion treatments, it is likely that the magnitude of the possible benefit of these LET effects is likely to be significantly less with protons. However, given previous results suggesting that protons may exhibit a higher RBE response for the same LET as compared to helium ions, further experiments are needed to fully assess the potential biological advantages of protons in treating tumors with lower photon radiosensitivities.

In addition to the effects of LET on the radiosensitivity of cancer cells, other physical factors such as fraction size may contribute to increased RBE values for protons in less radiosensitive cells. Although incompletely understood, these effects may be based on the relative flattening of the

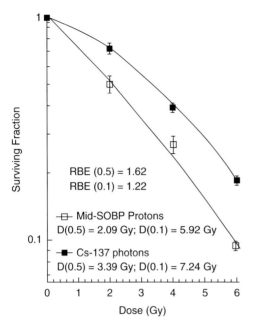

FIGURE 5
RBE values for 50% versus 10% surviving fraction. MSK-Leuk1 cells were irradiated using either ^{137}Cs photons or mid-SOBP protons from an R10.5M5 beam (SOBP with a maximal range of 10.5 cm with the final 5 cm modulated as an SOBP). D(0.1) and D(0.5) represent dose necessary to achieve 10% or 50% survival, respectively. RBE represents ratio of doses to achieve the indicated level of survival.

■ QUANTITATIVE AND QUALITATIVE DIFFERENCES IN DAMAGE TO CELLS

Alterations in Molecular Response to Radiation

Clonogenic cell survival measurements are a very important tool in studying the in vitro radiobiologic behavior of human cancer cells. The data appear to correlate well with the clinical radiation response of human tumors. More recently, significant insights have been gained into the cellular and molecular pathways that determine cellular radiosensitivity (14,27,28) and the interactions between tumor and normal tissues that lead to the malignant phenotype and altered tumor radiosensitivity (28,29). Recent data indicate that higher LET radiation may produce very different molecular responses in cancer cells as compared with photons, leading to the possibility that protons therapy may be uniquely suited for tumors with specific molecular lesions or phenotypes. The p53 pathway is one critical determinant of the cellular radiation response (27). Experiments with carbon ions suggest that high LET radiation can produce apoptosis in cancer cells that is independent of the cell's p53 mutational status (18,30,31). Studies in p53 mutant cancer cells suggest that protons have a high RBE, suggesting that protons may have a similar potential to produce p-53-independent cell death. In cells with wild-type p53, protons produce different gene expression profiles and are less efficient than photons at producing p53-dependent apoptosis in normal splenocytes, but may be more efficient at producing p53-dependent apoptosis in cancer cells (32–34).

Investigators at Loma Linda University found that proton radiation produced both qualitative and quantitative differences in the levels of micronucleus formation and apoptosis for the same radiation dose delivered as compared to gamma rays (35). In a continuation of these studies, these investigators found that the presence of connexin 32, a gap junction protein that promotes intercellular communication, was found to predict for

"shoulder" region of the survival curve for protons versus photons (Figure 5). The highest RBE values measured for protons appear to occur at lower fraction sizes (2–3 Gy), which correlate with surviving fractions of approximately greater than 50%. Using in vitro survival assays and V79 cells, several investigators have found increases in RBE from approximately 1.1 for doses producing less than 10% survival to 1.3 to 1.6 for proton doses producing 50% to 80% cell survival (23–26). In vivo, normal tissues such as lung, jejunum (small intestine), and testes showed no compelling evidence of fraction size variation in RBE (6,7,21,22).

decreased radiosensitivity to gamma rays but did not alter the proton radiosensitivity of Fischer rat thyroid cells (36). Taken together with previous findings that isolated cells in monolayer are often more radiosensitive than the same cells grown in a more organized tissue culture system (e.g., spheroids), these studies suggest that proton irradiation could be more useful than photons at overcoming tissue microenvironment-induced alterations in tumor radiosensitivity. However, protons may not improve the radiation responsiveness of cells with all molecular lesions or phenotypes. Preliminary evidence from the examination of the impact of the epidermal growth factor receptor (EGFR)/Ras radioresistance pathway suggests that proton radiotherapy may not provide a significant radiobiologic benefit in cells with highly activated EGFR/Ras signaling (KA Cengel, MJ Eblan, unpublished observations). In addition, protons have not shown evidence of improved response for highly hypoxic cells.

Risk of Second Malignancy with Protons

By delivering a lower integral body dose than photons, it is predicted that protons would produce a lower level of second malignant neoplasms (SMN) than photons (37). However, neutrons that can contaminate proton beams might increase the SMN risk to levels that are higher than predicted from considerations of integral body dose alone. Neutron contamination comes primarily from interaction of protons with high Z materials in the treatment head of the gantry. This effect is significantly worse with double scattered as opposed to scanned proton beams. A significantly small amount of neutron contamination of the proton beam also arises from interactions of protons in the patient's body. Estimates of SMN rates using older, currently outdated proton gantry designs have suggested that the SMN rate for these treatments would be much higher than the SMN rate for comparable IMRT-based photon treatments because of the higher levels of neutron

contamination (38,39). Using more modern double-scattering gantries, estimates of neutron production suggest that neutron contamination is about twofold higher for protons than IMRT within 25 cm of the field edge, but is two to threefold smaller outside of this distance (40–42). For scanning proton beams, neutron contamination is significantly smaller than either IMRT of passively scattered protons. While the neutron doses can be modeled with some accuracy for different forms of radiation therapy, the biological impact of these doses in terms of absolute increase in risk of SMN remains incompletely understood. Unfortunately, the long latency period for SMN induces a similarly long lag time in outcome data. Nevertheless, preliminary reports of proton SMN suggest that the rate of SMN for protons is, if anything, lower than the SMN rate for photon radiotherapy.

■ CONSIDERATIONS FOR EXPERIMENTAL DETERMINATION OF PROTON RBE

Methodologic Issues In Vitro

As described earlier, there is a significant difference in the range of RBE values reported using in vitro methods as compared to in vivo methods. Often the specific methods are not well described in the literature, but there are several areas where significant errors can be introduced that could under- or overestimate in vitro proton measured RBE. One source of error lies in the fact that most proton beam sources used for these experiments are in the form of a fixed horizontal beam, while most laboratory-based irradiators are in the form of a fixed vertical beam. This necessitates a change in irradiation setup that can lead to overestimation of proton RBE, especially at higher radiation doses (KA Cengel, A Rizzo, unpublished observations). Moreover, differences in temperature or other environmental conditions between the clinic and laboratory can affect cellular radiation response. Another potential source of this

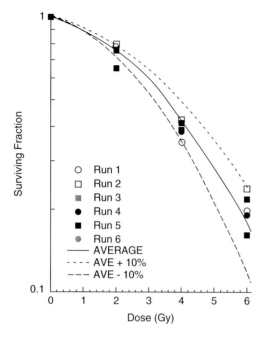

FIGURE 6

Clonogenic survival measurement variation over time. Results of six separate runs for clonogenic survival measurement of SQ20b head and neck squamous cell cancer cells treated with the indicated dose of ^{137}Cs photons are presented. Each data point represents the average ± standard deviation for replicate plates performed within the same run. Note that the spread on the data, which were collected over the course of several years, are contained within a 20% variation that from highest value to lowest values could be misinterpreted as an RBE of 1.2.

variation lies in comparing to "historical control" cell exposures. Over time, changes in the serum and culture conditions, laboratory personnel, and laboratory conditions can result in significant variation in the apparent radiosensitivity of any given cell line (Figure 6). Indeed, late passage cells (i.e., cells that have been growing in tissue culture for more than 20–30 generations) often have different radiosensitivity profiles that arise in part from alterations in the gene and molecular expression levels observed in these cells as compared to early

passage cells for the same cell line (36). Another source of variation is the "artificial" nature of the in vitro irradiation setup, where proton energies or other conditions can be tested on a tissue culture monolayer that does not exist in a meaningful way in vivo. However, it is important to note that in vivo experimental models are not without significant drawbacks and problems, as described in the following. In the end, therefore, the in vitro and in vivo evidence must be carefully weighed together prior to designing highly innovative new approaches to patient irradiation using proton beams.

Modeling the Effects of Stopping Beams in Humans Using Animals

When determining the RBE for protons for a specific organ, such as lung or bowel, a proton beam with an energy distribution that creates a homogenous dose distribution of protons (e.g., SOBP or plateau protons) can be compared to a parallel-opposed pair ^{60}Co beam arrangement. In this case, the high degree of similarity in overall dose distributions means that differences in biological effect are likely to represent true differences in RBE between these two forms of radiation. However, it is much more difficult to meaningfully compare the relatively homogenous ^{60}Co dose distributions to the proton dose distribution for proton beams that stop within the animal or beams that create a highly inhomogeneous dose distribution such as those now beginning to be employed in modern proton treatment planning to treat head and neck and other cancers. Preliminary preclinical evidence indicates that highly inhomogeneous dose distributions can have quantitatively and qualitatively different dose-response profiles for normal tissue irradiation (KA Cengel, AR Kennedy, unpublished observations). In making these comparisons of radiation forms with very different macroscopic dose distributions, it is considerably less clear whether any observed differences in absorbed dose response arise from differences in dose distribution or radiobiological effectiveness of protons versus ^{60}Co.

One way to solve this problem is to use electron beam radiation as the standard of comparison. Because of the intrinsic dose distribution pattern for MeV electrons, it is possible to reproduce the body distribution of proton radiation using a combination of different energy electrons. ^{60}Co deposits doses by scattering electrons in the MeV energy range. Thus, a primary electron beam in the MeV range has a nearly identical LET as ^{60}Co gamma rays and the RBE for electrons is defined as 1.0. Moreover, nearly 50 years worth of preclinical studies and more than 25 years of clinical experience have validated this assumption. Thus, comparisons of similar dose distributions of protons or other charged particles and electrons would help determine if an observed difference in radiobiologic response in comparison to ^{60}Co were due to differences in dose distribution or differences in the identity and nature of the particle. This technique is currently being employed in the study of the biological effects of whole body exposures to low energy protons (43).

Another added difficulty in these comparisons is whether to scale the energy of the protons to match the relative size difference between humans and small mammals such as mice. For a particular energy spectrum of protons used in humans to create a specific dose distribution or dose to specific organ systems of interest, a similar dose distribution or dose to specific organs can be created for use in a small animal model. However, because of the size (depth from beam entrance) differences between humans and laboratory animals, both the total radiation dose deposited as well as the distribution of this dose in tissues will be fundamentally different if the energy spectrum of the protons is kept constant from humans to animals.

The solution of "scaling down" the proton energy spectrum to account for these size differences to produce nearly equivalent dose distributions may alter the radiobiological characteristics of the proton beam. For example, 50 MeV protons treating a 30-cm diameter area of a human would need to be scaled down to 15 MeV protons in a mouse with diameter of 3 cm. While accounting for dose distribution, however, this method does not take into account the increase in the LET and RBE for protons used in the mouse experiments (Figure 2). Thus, by scaling the proton energy spectrum down to account for the smaller size of test animals compared with humans, the LET/RBE spectrum of the delivered protons increases significantly. Thus, there is a risk of dramatically overestimating the magnitude or possibly even the fundamental characteristics of the dose response. One way to manage this problem is to use large animal models. When testing the biological effects of protons in animals that are closer to human dimensions, the internal dose distribution can be reproduced between humans and animals with only minor energy scaling of protons. However, the tools and models for evaluating molecular and tumor-based endpoints that are frequently used in small animal models are not nearly as well developed in large animal models.

■ FUTURE DIRECTIONS

Chemoradiation with Protons and Cytotoxic/Molecularly Directed Therapies

There are currently limited preclinical data available on the response of tumor or normal tissues to combine modality treatment such as concurrent chemoradiotherapy, and clinical data are only beginning to emerge. One area that has received considerable attention lately is the interaction of high LET radiation with high Z chemotherapy (e.g., cisplatin). The theory behind the combination of platinum analogs with high LET radiation is that the increased local deposition of radiation dose due to interactions with high Z materials and the presence of two agents that are highly damaging to DNA will result in enhanced efficacy of chemoradiation as compared to photons.

Studies with carbon ions, helium ions, and fast neutrons using a variety of cell lines, including Chinese hamster ovary, murine lymphoma, and human glioblastoma cells, suggest that the enhancement of cell killing by platinum compounds is greater for high LET radiation than for photons and that these effects occur through a mechanism that involves increased damage to DNA (44–48). However, whether these effects could increase the cancer cell cytotoxicity of proton radiotherapy and the degree of cancer versus normal tissue specificity of this response remain unexplored. Of the molecularly targeted therapies that have been combined with radiotherapy to date, the combination of radiation with EGFR inhibitors has been the most successful. Studies are currently underway to determine the impact of activation or inhibition of EGFR pathway signaling on the proton radiosensitivity of cancer cells.

Scanned Beam Radiobiology

Scanning beam proton technologies represent an important part of the next generation of technological advancements in proton radiotherapy. Preliminary clinical evidence from Paul Scherrer Institute suggests that spot scanning can be performed safely and effectively in treatment of human cancers (49–51). One unexplored potential benefit of spot-scanned proton beams is the increased ability to specify the LET distribution for specific areas of tumor in addition to specifying only dose. If specific tumor areas or phenotypes could be identified in preclinical studies that might benefit from higher LET radiation, spot scanning could, in principle, be used to test the clinical potential of these findings. However, in order to realize this potential benefit, reduction in organ motion and patient setup uncertainties will likely be necessary, given the recent preclinical evidence shows increased variability of RBE measurements made with spot-scanned protons as compared with SOBP protons (52).

■ SUMMARY AND CONCLUSIONS

The spatial advantages of proton radiotherapy allows for increased dose to tumor as compared to normal tissues than conventional photon radiotherapy. Although the results for protons radiotherapy have largely corresponded well with previous photon radiotherapy experience, the assumption that proton radiobiology exactly mirrors photon radiobiology with a simple adjustment factor of 1.1 or 1.2 must be seen as a useful starting point approximation rather than a reason to stop actively studying proton radiobiology. Clearly, proton radiobiology needs to be re-examined in the light of the recent revolution in our understanding of the molecular mechanisms underlying the response of cells and tissues to ionizing radiation. In this way, the potential radiobiologic advantages of proton radiotherapy can be expanded to fully complement the spatial advantages and maximize therapeutic outcomes for patients.

■ REFERENCES

1. Gerweck LE, Kozin SV. Relative biological effectiveness of proton beams in clinical therapy. *Radiother Oncol.* 1999;50(2):135–142.
2. Paganetti H, Niemierko A, Ancukiewicz M, et al. Relative biological effectiveness (RBE) values for proton beam therapy. *Int J Radiat Oncol Biol Phys.* 2002; 53(2):407–421.
3. Slater JD. Clinical applications of proton radiation treatment at Loma Linda University: review of a fifteen-year experience. *Technol Cancer Res Treat.* 2006;5(2):81–89.
4. Weyrather WK, Debus J. Particle beams for cancer therapy. *Clin Oncol (R Coll Radiol).* 2003;15(1):S23–S28.
5. Stenerlöw B, Pettersson OA, Essand M, Blomquist E, Carlsson J. Irregular variations in radiation sensitivity when the linear energy transfer is increased. *Radiother Oncol.* 1995;36(2):133–142.
6. Tepper J, Verhey L, Goitein M, Suit HD. *In vivo* determinations of RBE in a high energy modulated proton beam using normal tissue reactions and fractionated dose schedules. *Int J Radiat Oncol Biol Phys.* 1977;2(11–12):1115–1122.
7. Urano M, Verhey LJ, Goitein M, et al. Relative biological effectiveness of modulated proton beams in

various murine tissues. *Int J Radiat Oncol Biol Phys.* 1984;10(4):509–514.

8. Belli M, Cera F, Cherubini R, et al. RBE-LET relationships for cell inactivation and mutation induced by low energy protons in V79 cells: further results at the LNL facility. *Int J Radiat Biol.* 1998;74(4): 501–509.

9. Paganetti H, Olko P, Kobus H, et al. Calculation of relative biological effectiveness for proton beams using biological weighting functions. *Int J Radiat Oncol Biol Phys.* 1997;37(3):719–729.

10. Tilly N, Johansson J, Isacsson U, et al. The influence of RBE variations in a clinical proton treatment plan for a hypopharynx cancer. *Phys Med Biol.* 2005; 50(12):2765–2777.

11. Eguchi-Kasai K, Murakami M, Itsukaichi H, et al. The role of DNA repair on cell killing by charged particles. *Adv Space Res.* 1996;18(1-2):109–118.

12. Suzuki M, Kase Y, Yamaguchi H, Kanai T, Ando K. Relative biological effectiveness for cell-killing effect on various human cell lines irradiated with heavy-ion medical accelerator in Chiba (HIMAC) carbon-ion beams. *Int J Radiat Oncol Biol Phys.* 2000; 48(1):241–250.

13. Weyrather WK, Ritter S, Scholz M, Kraft G. RBE for carbon track-segment irradiation in cell lines of differing repair capacity. *Int J Radiat Biol.* 1999; 75(11):1357–1364.

14. Cengel KA, McKenna WG. Molecular targets for altering radiosensitivity: lessons from Ras as a preclinical and clinical model. *Crit Rev Oncol Hematol.* 2005;55(2):103–116.

15. Tobias CA, Blakely EA, Chang PY, Lommel L, Roots R. Response of sensitive human ataxia and resistant T-1 cell lines to accelerated heavy ions. *Br J Cancer Suppl.* 1984;6:175–185.

16. Carlsson J, Stenerlöw B, Russell KR, Grusell E, Larsson B, Blomquist E. Cell type dependent effectiveness of tumour cell inactivation by radiation with increased ionisation density. *Anticancer Res.* 1995;15 (2):273–282.

17. Belli M, Bettega D, Calzolari P, et al. Inactivation of human normal and tumour cells irradiated with low energy protons. *Int J Radiat Biol.* 2000;76(6): 831–839.

18. Tsuchida Y, Tsuboi K, Ohyama H, Ohno T, Nose T, Ando K. Cell death induced by high-linear-energy transfer carbon beams in human glioblastoma cell lines. *Brain Tumor Pathol.* 1998;15(2):71–76.

19. Moertel H, Georgi JC, Distel L, et al. Effects of low energy protons on clonogenic survival, DSB repair and

cell cycle in human glioblastoma cells and B14 fibroblasts. *Radiother Oncol.* 2004;73(suppl 2):S115–S118.

20. Petrovic I, Ristic-Fira A, Todorovic D, Valastro L, Cirrone P, Cuttone G. Radiobiological analysis of human melanoma cells on the 62 MeV CATANA proton beam. *Int J Radiat Biol.* 2006;82(4):251–265.

21. Gueulette J, Böhm L, De Coster BM, et al. RBE variation as a function of depth in the 200-MeV proton beam produced at the National Accelerator Centre in Faure (South Africa). *Radiother Oncol.* 1997;42(3): 303–309.

22. Gueulette J, Bohm L, Slabbert JP, et al. Proton relative biological effectiveness (RBE) for survival in mice after thoracic irradiation with fractionated doses. *Int J Radiat Oncol Biol Phys.* 2000;47(4):1051–1058.

23. Wouters BG, Lam GK, Oelfke U, Gardey K, Durand RE, Skarsgard LD. Measurements of relative biological effectiveness of the 70 MeV proton beam at TRIUMF using Chinese hamster V79 cells and the high-precision cell sorter assay. *Radiat Res.* 1996;146(2):159–170.

24. Tang JT, Inoue T, Inoue T, et al. Comparison of radiobiological effective depths in 65-MeV modulated proton beams. *Br J Cancer.* 1997;76(2):220–225.

25. Blomquist E, Russell KR, Stenerlöw B, Montelius A, Grusell E, Carlsson J. Relative biological effectiveness of intermediate energy protons. Comparisons with 60Co gamma-radiation using two cell lines. *Radiother Oncol.* 1993;28(1):44–51.

26. Hall EJ, Kellerer AM, Rossi HH, Lam YM. The relative biological effectiveness of 160 MeV protons–II. Biological data and their interpretation in terms of microdosimetry. *Int J Radiat Oncol Biol Phys.* 1978; 4(11-12):1009–1013.

27. Lu C, El-Deiry WS. Targeting p53 for enhanced radio- and chemo-sensitivity. *Apoptosis.* 2009;14(4):597–606.

28. Karar J, Maity A. Modulating the tumor microenvironment to increase radiation responsiveness. *Cancer Biol Ther.* 2009;8(21):1994–2001.

29. Giaccia AJ, Schipani E. Role of carcinoma-associated fibroblasts and hypoxia in tumor progression. *Curr Top Microbiol Immunol.* 2010;810:31–45.

30. Iwadate Y, Mizoe J, Osaka Y, Yamaura A, Tsujii H. High linear energy transfer carbon radiation effectively kills cultured glioma cells with either mutant or wild-type p53. *Int J Radiat Oncol Biol Phys.* 2001; 50(3):803–808.

31. Mori E, Takahashi A, Yamakawa N, Kirita T, Ohnishi T. High LET heavy ion radiation induces p53-independent apoptosis. *J Radiat Res.* 2009;50(1):37–42.

32. Finnberg N, Wambi C, Ware JH, Kennedy AR, El-Deiry WS. Gamma-radiation (GR) triggers a unique

gene expression profile associated with cell death compared to proton radiation (PR) in mice in vivo. *Cancer Biol Ther.* 2008;7(12):2023–2033.

33. Ghosh S, Bhat NN, Santra S, et al. Low energy proton beam induces efficient cell killing in A549 lung adenocarcinoma cells. *Cancer Invest.* 2010;28 (6):615–622.

34. Lee KB, Kim KR, Huh TL, Lee YM. Proton induces apoptosis of hypoxic tumor cells by the p53-dependent and p38/JNK MAPK signaling pathways. *Int J Oncol.* 2008;33(6):1247–1256.

35. Green LM, Murray DK, Bant AM, et al. Response of thyroid follicular cells to gamma irradiation compared to proton irradiation. I. Initial characterization of DNA damage, micronucleus formation, apoptosis, cell survival, and cell cycle phase redistribution. *Radiat Res.* 2001;155(1 Pt 1):32–42.

36. Green LM, Tran DT, Murray DK, Rightnar SS, Todd S, Nelson GA. Response of thyroid follicular cells to gamma irradiation compared to proton irradiation: II. The role of connexin 32. *Radiat Res.* 2002;158(4):475–485.

37. Miralbell R, Lomax A, Cella L, Schneider U. Potential reduction of the incidence of radiation-induced second cancers by using proton beams in the treatment of pediatric tumors. *Int J Radiat Oncol Biol Phys.* 2002;54(3):824–829.

38. Hall EJ. Intensity-modulated radiation therapy, protons, and the risk of second cancers. *Int J Radiat Oncol Biol Phys.* 2006;65(1):1–7.

39. Hall EJ. The impact of protons on the incidence of second malignancies in radiotherapy. *Technol Cancer Res Treat.* 2007;6(4 suppl):31–34.

40. Athar BS, Bednarz B, Seco J, Hancox C, Paganetti H. Comparison of out-of-field photon doses in 6 MV IMRT and neutron doses in proton therapy for adult and pediatric patients. *Phys Med Biol.* 2010; 55(10):2879–2891.

41. Paganetti H. Nuclear interactions in proton therapy: dose and relative biological effect distributions originating from primary and secondary particles. *Phys Med Biol.* 2002;47(5):747–764.

42. Paganetti H, Bortfeld T, Delaney TF. Neutron dose in proton radiation therapy: in regard to Eric J. Hall (Int J Radiat Oncol Biol Phys 2006;65:1-7). *Int J Radiat*

Oncol Biol Phys. 2006;66(5):1594-1595; author reply 1595.

43. Cengel KA, Diffenderfer ES, Avery S, et al. Using electron beam radiation to simulate the dose distribution for whole body solar particle event proton exposure. *Radiat Environ Biophys.* 2010. [Epub ahead of print]

44. Benzina S, Altmeyer A, Malek F, et al. High-LET radiation combined with oxaliplatin induce autophagy in U-87 glioblastoma cells. *Cancer Lett.* 2008;264(1):63–70.

45. Fischer B, Benzina S, Ganansia-Leymarie V, et al. Cisplatin enhances the cytotoxicity of fast neutrons in a murine lymphoma cell line. *Can J Physiol Pharmacol.* 2004;82(2):140–145.

46. Usami N, Furusawa Y, Kobayashi K, et al. Fast He2+ion irradiation of DNA loaded with platinum-containing molecules. *Int J Radiat Biol.* 2005;81(7):515–522.

47. Usami N, Furusawa Y, Kobayashi K, et al. Mammalian cells loaded with platinum-containing molecules are sensitized to fast atomic ions. *Int J Radiat Biol.* 2008; 84(7):603–611.

48. Usami N, Kobayashi K, Furusawa Y, et al. Irradiation of DNA loaded with platinum containing molecules by fast atomic ions C6+and Fe26+. *Int J Radiat Biol.* 2007;83(9):569–576.

49. Timmermann B, Schuck A, Niggli F, et al. Spot-scanning proton therapy for malignant soft tissue tumors in childhood: first experiences at the Paul Scherrer Institute. *Int J Radiat Oncol Biol Phys.* 2007;67(2):497–504.

50. Weber DC, Lomax AJ, Rutz HP, et al.; Swiss Proton Users Group. Spot-scanning proton radiation therapy for recurrent, residual or untreated intracranial meningiomas. *Radiother Oncol.* 2004;71(3):251–258.

51. Weber DC, Rutz HP, Pedroni ES, et al. Results of spot-scanning proton radiation therapy for chordoma and chondrosarcoma of the skull base: the Paul Scherrer Institute experience. *Int J Radiat Oncol Biol Phys.* 2005;63(2):401–409.

52. Gueulette J, Blattmann H, Pedroni E, et al. Relative biologic effectiveness determination in mouse intestine for scanning proton beam at Paul Scherrer Institute, Switzerland. Influence of motion. *Int J Radiat Oncol Biol Phys.* 2005;62(3):838–845.

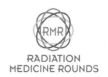

RADIATION
MEDICINE ROUNDS

The Need for and Future of Clinical Studies of Proton Therapy

John P. Christodouleas* and Stephen M. Hahn

University of Pennsylvania School of Medicine, Philadelphia, PA

■ ABSTRACT

Demographic changes are driving an increasing demand for proton therapy (PT). At the same time, there is a growing political and medical imperative to show that this emerging technology produces a measurable benefit to our patients with cancer. This review finds that the published clinical evidence in support of PT is currently limited and the vast majority of the existing papers describe retrospective and single-institution studies. However, the future is promising as the number of clinical studies is increasing and important clinical research infrastructural improvements are underway. In addition, because PT indications and techniques are rapidly evolving, traditional phase-based clinical research studies will need to be complemented by alternative research strategies. This review suggests that procedure registries may be particularly useful for studying PT.

Keywords: proton therapy, clinical studies, clinical research, procedure registry

■ INTRODUCTION

Proton therapy (PT) is a promising emerging technology. Clinical studies, ones that assess patient outcomes, will play an important role in defining how PT emerges. The goals of this chapter are, first, to describe the growing demand for clinical studies of PT; second, summarize the current level of evidence in support for PT; and third, describe future approaches to PT's clinical evaluation.

■ CLINICAL STUDIES OF THE VALUE OF PT ARE IMPERATIVE

The Increasing Demand for and Availability of PT

Demographic changes in the United States are driving a dramatic increase in the need for radiation

*Corresponding author, Department of Radiation Oncology, University of Pennsylvania School of Medicine, Philadelphia, PA

E-mail address: christojo@uphs.upenn.edu

Radiation Medicine Rounds 1:3 (2010) 455–470.
DOI: 10.5003/2151–4208.1.3.455

treatment: the vast majority of all cancers are diagnosed in people older than 60 years of age, an age group expected to increase in size by 33% between 2010 and 2020 (1). Dovetailing with the growth in demand for radiation treatments generally and PT in particular is a significant increase in PT availability. The first hospital based-PT center in the United States began treating patients in 1990, and only two additional facilities opened over the next 15 years. In 2005, PT represented less than 1% of all annual radiation treatments. Beginning in 2005, PT facilities began opening in earnest, and currently there are seven of them, all of which are large, multiroom treatment centers. An additional three multiroom PT centers are in the construction phase and are due to open in the next 12 to 18 months for a total of 10 multiroom centers by the end of 2012. A similar growth in PT utilization is occurring abroad. Currently, there are 24 multiroom PT centers operating outside of the United States. Another 18 centers are expected to be operational by 2012.

However, much of the technology included in FDA-approved PT systems dates from 20 years ago and does not reflect technology advances that have proven effective in research laboratories. More recent technological innovations are already being introduced in new PT centers and may revolutionize PT delivery and significantly reduce its cost over the next 5 to 10 years. One such innovation is the recent development of single-room PT systems. Although all of these systems are still in initial testing, at least 17 U.S. hospitals have already indicated interest in such single-room PT systems. Other technologies under development have the potential of greatly reducing the cost of building PT centers. Smaller and cheaper PT systems would allow for a more uniform geographic distribution of PT centers and could result in a dramatic increase in PT utilization. Today there are approximately 2,300 x-ray linear accelerators operating in the United States with a replacement cycle of about 8 years. It is quite possible that in 10 years a significant proportion of these replacements will be proton facilities.

Not only will the absolute number of PT treatments increase in the United States, but the setting in which it is applied will shift away from academic tertiary care centers to community centers. Prior to 2009, all PT centers in the United States and abroad were affiliated with and funded by academic tertiary care centers. In 2009, the first community-based PT center began treating patients in Oklahoma City. At least four additional large, multiroom, community-based PT centers are either under construction or are far along in the development process (2). This change in setting could also have an important impact on the way PT is used over the next decade.

The Increasing Demand for Evidence

Currently, PT treatments come at a substantial financial cost. Although estimates vary, the up-front cost of building a multiroom PT center range from 2 to 10 times the cost of building a similarly sized x-ray radiation facility. In addition, Medicare currently pays about 40% more for PT than for comparable x-ray treatment. Therefore, as PT emerges the potential for cost-ineffective uses of PT are significant, and health care payers are aware of this.

Historically, many new technologies have been adopted into the radiation oncology clinic prior to rigorous evaluation in prospective clinical studies. Consider intensity-modulated radiation therapy (IMRT), for example. A pattern of care survey by Mell et al. found that IMRT adoption among American radiation oncologists increased from 32% in 2002 to 63% in 2004. This occurred at a time when the benefits of IMRT were mostly considered theoretical as long-term outcome data with IMRT were lacking (3).

The adoption of IMRT reflects a paradigm that may no longer be relevant in radiation oncology. That paradigm was based on a presumption that health care payers would cover technologies that have been shown to be safe. The burden on physicians and manufacturers to establish efficacy focused primarily on short-term outcomes.

However, there is evidence suggesting that the perspective of payers is changing, particularly that of the Centers for Medicare and Medicaid Services (CMS). In 2000, CMS clarified the primary factors involved in its national determinations of what technologies would be covered. It made clear its interest in covering technologies not only shown to be safe but also substantially medically beneficial or otherwise value-adding, for instance, by providing an alternative treatment modality to its covered population (4). Indeed, a review of all complete national coverage determinations (NCDs) between 1999 and 2008 suggests that the CMS has become more critical of the data that support new treatments (5). In these NCDs, the evidence supporting a therapy/technology has been increasingly criticized for lack of relevant outcomes, data applicability to Medicare populations, and lack of blinding.

More evidence of the heightened emphasis on evidence comes from federal legislative initiatives. In 2009, the U.S. Congress passed the American Recovery and Reinvestment Act, which included US $1.1 billion commitment toward comparative-effectiveness research in health care. In 2010, the U.S. Congress passed a comprehensive national health care reform package, the Affordable Care Act, which established an independent panel of medical experts (the Independent Payment Advisory Board [IPAB]) charged with making changes to Medicare's payment system. Starting in 2014, if Medicare's per capita costs exceed a predefined threshold, the IPAB must institute policies for reducing this excess. By law, these policies are in force, up until the time Congress passes alternative policies that result in the same savings. This rule, and the structure with which it is enforced, will create powerful pressures on Medicare to endorse only those technologies with clearly established clinical value (6).

Certainly, these political and societal pressures will motivate the PT community to produce data showing the value of PT. More important, however, is the medical imperative to show that this emerging technology produces a measurable benefit to our patients with cancer. Providers of PT should expect to provide more comprehensive outcomes data to meet these obligations.

■ PUBLISHED CLINICAL STUDIES OF PT ARE LIMITED

The Current Available Evidence

Although a large number of papers on PT have been published, the vast majority of them are nonclinical, that is, dosimetric or planning studies. According to a systematic review by Trikalinos et al., only 126 papers reporting patient outcomes with PT have been published (as of the end of 2007) (7). The vast majority of these describe retrospective, single-arm institutional series. These papers address the feasibility of using PT in a number of cancer types: pediatric CNS, low-grade glioma, meningioma, adenoid cystic, uveal melanoma, bone and soft-tissue sarcomas, esophagus, breast, non–small cell lung, primary liver, cervix, bladder, and prostate. However, clinical studies that compare PT to alternative modalities are even rarer. Only seven comparative studies have been published, and they involved only uveal melanoma (four) (8–11) and prostate cancer (three) (12–14). Only one of these comparative studies was randomized (14).

Comparative Studies in Uveal Melanoma

The effectiveness of PT compared to enucleation in the treatment of uveal melanoma was evaluated in two papers from the Massachusetts Eye and Ear Infirmary. Seddon et al., (9,11) published uveal melanoma outcomes for their patients in 1985 and 1990. The second paper included a greater number of patients and longer follow-up of their cohort. In both papers, the authors retrospectively compared disease-specific and overall survival after PT versus enucleation and concluded that treatment choice had little influence on survival outcomes. Although these studies did not provide randomized evidence, they did help establish organ preservation with PT as safe choice for selected uveal melanoma patients.

Two subsequent studies have compared outcomes of PT and plaque brachytherapy for uveal melanoma. In 1999, Wilson MQ and Hungerford JL reported outcomes for uveal melanoma patients treated with PT, iodine 125 plaque brachytherapy, and ruthenium-106 plaque brachytherapy. Based on a retrospective analysis, it was found that local recurrence was worse in patients treated with ruthenium-106 brachytherapy but similar in patients treated with PT and iodine 125 brachytherapy. A similar study in 2003, Desjardins et al., included 1,272 uveal melanoma patients and retrospectively compared local recurrence after PT against iodine 125 plaque brachytherapy (8). After a median follow-up of 5 years, there was no significant difference in local recurrence rate between the two procedures. It should be noted, however, that the brachytherapy procedure was typically only used in more easily accessible anterior tumors whereas posterior tumors were treated with PT.

The aforementioned studies suggest that PT has an important role in uveal melanoma, though a significant subset of patients can also be adequately treated with iodine 125 plaque brachytherapy. Nonetheless, even in the case of uveal melanoma, which has been relatively well studied, PT has not been evaluated in the setting of a randomized trial.

Comparative Studies in Prostate Cancer

The role of PT in prostate cancer is discussed in detail in a separate chapter in this issue. Here we briefly summarize the three comparative studies involving PT in the treatment of prostate cancer.

In the oldest comparative study, published in 1983, Duttenhaver et al., retrospectively evaluated 116 prostate cancer patients treated with two-dimensional x-ray therapy at Massachusetts General Hospital (MGH) between 1972 and 1979 (13). As many as 64 of these men received a PT-based tumor boost. Authors reported no difference in treatment morbidity, nor did they report any difference in cancer-control outcomes, even though follow-up was limited. This study served as the foundation of a subsequent randomized trial at MGH that compared men treated with x-ray therapy to 67.2 Gy or with mixed x-ray and PT to 75.6 Gy (14). Authors reported that the chances of survival did not improve with the PT boost, including 8-year overall survival, disease-specific survival, or total recurrence-free survival. In addition, rectal bleeding was significantly worse in the PT boost arm. Eight years is probably not adequate follow-up to show anything but very large differences in major cancer-control outcomes for prostate cancer, so it is not surprising that this randomized trial was negative. However, even if the results did favor the PT boost arm, the study would no longer be relevant. Since the publication of this study 15 years ago, numerous studies have shown that more advanced x-ray-based treatments (3D conformal and IMRT) can be used to safely treat prostate cancer patients to total doses of 75.6 Gy and higher.

In a more recent paper from 2001, Galbraith et al., report a nonrandomized longitudinal study of health-related quality of life and health status in 185 prostate cancer patients treated with watchful waiting, prostatectomy, x-ray radiation, PT, and mixed x-ray and PT (12). The study used surveys that were completed at 6, 12, and 18 months after enrollment. The authors found no significant differences in health-related quality of life or health status by treatment. Given the small number of patients in each treatment cohort and the limited follow-up, this study was likely powered only to show very large differences in health-related quality of life and health status.

The Number of Clinical Studies Is Increasing

To our knowledge, the seven studies discussed earlier represent the entire body of clinical studies that compare PT to an alternative therapy. These studies have numerous individual shortcomings, but the major limitation with the literature overall is simply that not enough work has been done. If taxpayers will require clinical comparative studies to firmly establish the value of PT, that evidence does not yet exist.

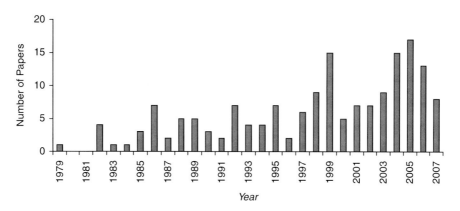

FIGURE 1
The data in this figure were derived from a systematic review by Trikalinos et al. (7). That review included all PT clinical studies that included 10 or more patients published in English, German, French, Italian, and Japanese and were available in MEDLINE from 1950 to 2008.

With the increasing availability of PT, however, there are clear signs that clinical studies are also increasing. Figure 1 shows the number of comparative and noncomparative clinical studies of PT by publication year and reflects a growing body of research.

In addition, there are already a large number of ongoing clinical studies internationally and nationally. Table 1 summarizes all of the active (completed or accruing) PT-related trials by institutional sponsor and disease site as listed with the National Cancer Institute (NCI) as of July 18, 2010.

The Research Infrastructure for Multi-institutional Clinical Studies of PT Is Improving

The past several years have seen important progress in the infrastructure required to evaluate PT in multi-institutional clinical-trial cooperatives. One issue that complicates the use of PT in the cooperative groups is the lack of credentialing and quality-assurance (QA) procedures. The NCI has recently addressed this by providing guidelines for the use of PT in NCI-sponsored cooperative group trials (15). One of the requirements of these guidelines is that sites be credentialed by a QA center that will be designated by each protocol. Although criteria for credentialing do not yet exist, the Advanced Technology Consortium (ATC), an organization that provides QA support for NCI-sponsored clinical trials, is actively developing the credentialing criteria. In addition, the Radiation Therapy Oncology Group (RTOG), through its proton working group, is cultivating clinical trials that will include PT in anticipation that credentialing procedures will be fully formulated in the near future (Jeff Michalski and Tom Delaney, personal communication, July 2010).

Of note, the pediatric cooperative groups began to allow PT in 1997 when the Intergroup Rhabdomyosarcoma Study Group (IRSG) included it in their low-risk rhabdomyosarcoma protocol. From that time forward, PT has been included in protocols for pediatric sarcoma, including the current studies of the Children's Oncology Group (COG), and the Pediatric

TABLE 1
Active clinical studies of PT

Sponsor	Study Title
	CNS
MDACC	Phase II evaluation of proton beam therapy for skull base chondrosarcoma
	Phase II randomized trial of 70 Gy versus 78 Gy proton beam therapy for skull base chordoma
MGH	Late effects of proton radiation therapy in patients with low-grade glioma
	Phase II study of craniospinal and posterior fossa irradiation using proton beam radiotherapy for medulloblastoma and pineoblastoma: assessment of acute and long-term sequelae
	Phase II study of proton radiation therapy for CNS germ cell tumors: evaluation of acute and late side effects
	Hypoxia-PET and intensity-modulated proton therapy dose painting in patients with chordomas: a pilot study
	Proton beam radiotherapy for medulloblastoma and pineoblastoma: an assessment of acute toxicity and long-term neurocognitive, neuroendocrine, and ototoxicity outcomes
	Pituitary adenoma
	Chordomas and chondrosarcomas
UFPTI	Clinical outcomes study of proton radiation therapy for pituitary adenoma
	A clinical outcomes protocol of proton beam radiation therapy for chordomas and/or chondrosarcomas of the base of skull and/or spine
	A study of late effects after proton radiotherapy for pediatric tumors of the brain, head, and neck
	Risk-adapted therapy for children less than 3 years of age with embryonal brain tumors, high-grade glioma, choroid plexus carcinoma, or ependymoma
UPenn	Proton beam radiation therapy in treating patients with low grade gliomas
	Proton beam radiation for WHO grade I/III meningiomas and hemangiopericytomas
	Cervix
UPenn	A feasibility and phase II study of proton beam radiotherapy for patients with cervical cancer and FDG-PET positive para-aortic lymph nodes
	Head and neck
MGH	A phase II study of proton radiotherapy with chemotherapy for nasopharyngeal carcinoma
UFPTI	A clinical outcomes protocol of photon/proton beam radiation therapy for cancers of the nasal cavity and/or paranasal sinuses
	A clinical outcomes protocol of photon/proton beam radiation therapy for oropharyngeal cancers
	A clinical outcomes protocol of photon/proton beam radiation therapy for carcinoma of the nasopharynx
	A clinical outcomes protocol of photon/proton beam radiation therapy for carcinoma of the skin of the head and neck with perineural invasion
UPenn	A feasibility and phase I dose escalation study of proton beam radiotherapy for locally advanced nasopharyngeal squamous cell carcinoma
	Ocular
MDACC	A phase II trial of proton beam radiation therapy for intra- and periocular retinoblastoma
UCDavis	Pilot study of lucentis combined with proton beam irradiation in treating wet age-related macular degeneration

Continued

TABLE 1
Active clinical studies of PT   (*Continued*)

Sponsor	Study Title
	Breast
LLU	Phase II trial of lumpectomy and partial breast proton therapy for early stage breast cancer
	Lymphoma
UFPTI	Improving the therapeutic ratio by using proton beam radiation therapy for patients with stage IA-IIIBX (bulky/nonbulky) Hodgkin lymphoma involving the mediastinum following standard chemotherapy
	Lung
LLU	Phase I/II study of combined chemotherapy and high dose, accelerated proton radiation for the treatment of locally advanced non–small cell lung carcinoma
MDACC	Phase II concurrent proton and chemotherapy in locally advanced stage IIIA/B non–small cell lung cancer (NSCLC)
	Phase II escalated/accelerated proton radiotherapy for inoperable stage I (T1-T2, N0, M0) and selected stage II (T3N0M0) NSCLC
	A Bayesian randomized trial of image-guided adaptive conformal photon versus proton therapy, with concurrent chemotherapy, for locally advanced non–small cell lung carcinoma: treatment related pneumonitis and locoregional recurrence
UFPTI	A phase II trial of three-dimensional proton radiotherapy with concomitant chemotherapy for patients with initially unresectable stage III NSCLC
	Hypofractionated, image-guided radiation therapy with proton therapy for stage I NSCLC
UPenn	Phase I dose escalation trial of proton beam radiotherapy with concurrent chemotherapy and nelfinavir for inoperable stage III NSCLC
	Feasibility and phase I/II trial of preoperative proton beam radiotherapy with concurrent chemotherapy for resectable stage IIIA or superior sulcus NSCLC
	Esophagus
MDACC	Oxaliplatin-based chemotherapy and chemoradiotherapy or chemoradiotherapy in esophageal or gastroesophageal carcinoma
	Liver
LLU	Proton beam therapy for treatment of hepatocellular carcinoma
	Randomized controlled trial of transarterial chemoembolization versus proton beam radiotherapy for the treatment of hepatocellular carcinoma
MDACC	Phase I study of proton radiotherapy and bevacizumab for primary liver tumors
MGH	Proton beam irradiation for the treatment of unresectable hepatocellular cancer or hepatic metastases
	Phase II study of proton beam irradiation for the treatment of unresectable hepatocellular cancer and cholangiocarcinoma
	Pancreas
MGH	Phase I/II of neoadjuvant accelerated short course radiation therapy with proton beam and capecitabine for resectable pancreatic cancer
UFPTI	A pilot study using neoadjuvant proton beam radiation therapy and chemotherapy for marginally resectable carcinoma of the pancreas
	A study using photon/proton beam radiation therapy and chemotherapy for unresectable carcinoma of the pancreas

Continued

TABLE 1
Active clinical studies of PT (*Continued*)

Sponsor	Study Title
	Prostate
LLU	Phase I/II trial of hypofractionated conformal proton beam radiation therapy for favorable-risk prostate cancer
MDACC	Prospective evaluation of quality of life after proton therapy for prostate cancer
UFPTI	A phase II study of hypofractionated image guided proton radiation therapy for low and intermediate risk adenocarcinoma of the prostate
	Semen analysis following definitive treatment of prostate cancer with proton therapy alone
	A phase II study of proton-based radiation therapy with elective pelvic nodal irradiation, concomitant docetaxel, and adjuvant androgen deprivation for high-risk prostate adenocarcinoma
	Postoperative or salvage radiotherapy for node negative prostate cancer following radical prostatectomy
UPenn	A feasibility trial of proton radiation therapy using standard fractionation for low-risk adenocarcinoma of the prostate
	A feasibility trial of proton radiation with mild hypofractionation for intermediate risk adenocarcinoma of the prostate
	Bone and sarcoma
MGH	Proton radiation for the treatment of pediatric bone and nonrhabdomyosarcoma soft tissue sarcomas
	A phase II trial of proton RT for the treatment of pediatric rhabdomyosarcoma
UFPTI	A pilot study investigating preoperative proton radiotherapy for retroperitoneal sarcoma
	A pilot study investigating neoadjuvant temozolomide-based proton chemoradiotherapy for high-risk soft tissue sarcomas
UPenn	Proton radiation for chordomas and chondrosarcomas
	Proton radiotherapy for retroperitoneal sarcoma
	Proton radiotherapy for extremity soft tissue sarcoma
	Retreatment
UPenn	Retreatment of recurrent tumors using proton radiotherapy

Abbreviations: LLU, Loma Linda University Medical Center; MDACC, MD Anderson Cancer Center; MGH, Massachusetts General Hospital; UCD, University of California at Davis; UFPTI, University of Florida Proton Therapy Institute; UPENN, University of Pennsylvania

Source: www.clinicaltrials.gov. Accessed July 18, 2010.

Cooperative Group, which was formed when the IRSG, the Pediatric Oncology Group (POG), and the Children's Cancer Study Group (CCSG) merged in 2000. The earliest use of PT in pediatric brain tumor trials dates from 2000 when it was first allowed in a medulloblastoma study, COG A9934. With a few exceptions, most new and current studies of pediatric sarcoma and CNS tumors include PT and adhere to NCI guidelines, save for the requirement that centers be credentialed; however, this requirement is being deferred until consensus credentialing processes are finalized (Tom Merchant, personal communication, July 2010).

In addition, a new clinical trials cooperative group dedicated exclusively to studies of PT has been proposed. This organization, called the Proton Collaborative Group (PCG), is currently in the process of developing its infrastructure but appears to be on track to open multi-institutional trials by 2011.

■ MULTIPLE RESEARCH STRATEGIES ARE BEING PURSUED

In the previous section, we showed that despite currently limited evidence in support of PT, there is a clear and promising trend toward increasing evidence development. In this section, we discuss different research strategies for clarifying the role of PT.

The Role of Randomized Trials of PT

Between 2005 and 2007, several systematic reviews of the clinical evidence for PT were published, one of which concluded that "an uncontrolled expansion of clinical units offering as yet unproven and expensive PT is unlikely to advance the field of radiation oncology or be a benefit to cancer patients" (16). This review and others prompted a series of editorials discussing how best to evaluate the role of PT. In a provocative editorial in the *Journal of Clinical Oncology* in 2008, Goiten and Cox argued that randomized studies would likely have only a limited role in establishing the role of PT because practitioners of PT lack equipoise in many clinical scenarios (17). The authors argued an absence of equipoise because (a) the dose distributions that can be achieved with protons are in almost all cases better than those possible with x-rays, (b) there is virtually no difference in tissue response per unit dose between protons of therapeutic energies and x-rays, and (c) increased radiation doses to normal tissues causes increased damage. Goitein and Cox write: "It is therefore hard to imagine how any objective person could avoid the conclusion that there is, at the very least, a high probability that protons can provide superior therapy to that possible with x-rays in almost all circumstances." As such, they contend that many of the studies of PT will involve determining not whether there is a benefit, but rather the degree of benefit. For these kinds of questions, the argument goes that randomized trials are not the appropriate study design, as it would be unethical to randomize a patient to a study arm one expects to be inferior.

There have been numerous responses to Goitein and Cox's editorial that generally have made the case for a more expansive role for randomized studies in evaluating PT (18–20). This can be summarized as follows: (a) The delivery of cancer therapy is a highly complex clinical situation in which the modeled dose distribution is only one of many clinical parameters, thus making it hard to accurately predict which parameters actually have any impact on relevant clinical outcomes; (b) because of the substantial costs associated with PT, we have a societal obligation to confirm PT's value; and (c) the most rigorous way to confirm PT's value, given the clinical complexities involved, is via randomized studies.

Whereas the disagreements in these editorials have garnered much attention in the field of radiation oncology, our view is that the differences between the authors on either side of the argument are largely, though not exclusively, semantic: One person's "limited role" may be another person's "expansive role." When one considers concrete clinical scenarios, it is likely that both the promoters and detractors of randomization will agree on the actual role of randomization (though not necessarily on the value of PT). Consider the example of standard-risk medulloblastoma, a disease with a median age of diagnosis of approximately 6 years but which is associated with long-term survival rates near 80% (21). With increasing availability of treatment facilities providing PT, the use of PT in medulloblastoma is growing. However, published clinical outcomes of PT in medulloblastoma are limited to the short-term outcome of only four patients (22). The expected advantages of PT over photon therapy are purely based on radiation-planning studies. Nonetheless, not even the most ardent advocates of randomization would likely argue that PT's comparative efficacy in medulloblastoma should be confirmed by a randomized trial. In the case of medulloblastoma, the planning studies are so compelling and the potential impact on health care costs so small (due to the rarity of the disease) that most radiation oncologists would likely agree that, when available, PT should be the treatment of choice. Similarly, there are also clinical scenarios where the need for randomization is more obvious, that is, scenarios in which there are clear tradeoffs between modalities. In our view, a good example is locally advanced non–small cell lung cancer, a common disease for which the dosimetric advantages of PT may be outweighed by the considerable uncertainties associated with PT and lung motion (23). Indeed, two leading PT centers are already accruing to a phase II clinical study on locally advanced non–small cell lung cancer that includes randomization. It is worth noting that the two institutions involved in this important study are also the homes of Drs. Goitein and Cox, whose concerns about randomized studies sparked so much debate. We anticipate that, as a practical matter, most practitioners of PT will largely agree on which clinical scenarios randomization is ethically appropriate.

Of course, even when the ethics of randomization are not controversial, there may be other reasonable arguments against attempting a randomized study. Our institution recently participated in the submission of a multi-institutional proposal for a randomized trial of PT versus photon therapy for low-risk prostate cancer. In the development phase of this study, a number of investigators argued that a randomized trial was not the appropriate study design, but their concern was not an ethical one. These investigators were concerned about the feasibility of randomizing low-risk prostate cancer patients, many of whom come in to consultations at proton centers with strong biases for PT. In this case, our research group ultimately decided that randomization was feasible. Yet these kinds

of practical concerns can be legitimate arguments against attempting a randomized trial of PT.

Registries as a Complement to Traditional Phase-By-Phase Clinical Studies

Before phase III randomized trials can be designed, it is critical that a clear understanding of expected outcomes be determined though rigorous cohort studies. This is best done through prospective (phase II) studies whose treatments and outcomes are similar to the ones that will be used in the subsequent phase III trial. As discussed earlier, the vast majority of PT studies so far have been retrospective in design. As such, there is a critical need for high-quality phase II studies. The use of PT to treat solid malignancies with combined chemoradiotherapy is relatively unexplored and deserves further study. Hypofractionated treatment schedules and combined proton–photon treatment regimens are also important examples of future phase II studies. Table 1 shows that many of these are ongoing. However, traditional phase-based clinical studies (PBCSs) may have important limitations in the evaluation of PT. As discussed earlier, PT is a rapidly evolving technology, and there may be dramatic changes in both the frequency of its use and the types of scenarios in which it is used. The sheer number of technical questions to be studied and the high time and financial costs of PBCSs necessitate alternative strategies for studying PT. The emergence of PT requires a strategy that provides a real-time description of utilization and robust outcomes estimates for these uses so that effective and ineffective uses of PT can be rapidly identified. These needs may be met by registry studies.

Although there is no consensus definition of a registry study (24), we will use it here to refer to a study that is prospective and observational, has broad inclusion criteria with respect to the kinds of patients enrolled and the kinds of treatments given, and explicitly tracks only a limited number of outcomes.

It is instructive to highlight three emergent features of registries. First, in contrast to retrospective cohort studies, registries use uniform data collection procedures and data definitions for every patient. For example, a registry of PT in localized prostate cancer may provide a uniform definition of rectal bleeding, say rectal bleeding involving 3 or more occurrences over 2 or more weeks, so that rectal bleeding estimates do not vary by treating physician because of different thresholds for scoring rectal bleeding. Thus, registries may minimize or eliminate many of the biases inherent in retrospective studies, such as recall or interpretation biases. Second, registries include relatively heterogeneous cohorts compared to PBCSs that, in contrast, attempt to minimize confounders by minimizing heterogeneity. For example, a registry of PT in locally advanced non–small cell lung cancer might enroll both stage IIIA and IIIB patients and allow a range of total treatment doses, say 60 to 80 Gy. A PBCSS, on the other hand, would typically include either stage IIIA or IIIB and narrowly define the treatment technique and total doses used. In this way, the results of registry studies may be more prone to confounding than those of PBCSs. Third, registries are typically less expensive to run on a per-patient basis than PBCSs because they are broadly inclusive and track only a limited number of outcomes.

Thus, registries are good vehicles for research questions that require large cohorts, such as verifying treatment outcomes in different regions of the country or performing utilization reviews.

■ THE STUDY OF PT WOULD BENEFIT FROM A NATIONALLY REPRESENTATIVE PROCEDURE REGISTRY

In order to optimize the emergence of PT (maximize the use of effective treatments and minimize the use of ineffective treatments), registry studies will be needed to compliment PBCSs. We propose a procedure registry below called the Adaptive Proton Therapy (APT) registry, in which multiple institutions with PT capabilities would attempt to enroll every patient treated (either PT or photon). APT would provide a real-time description of PT utilization and robust cancer-control and toxicity estimates so that effective and ineffective uses of PT could be rapidly identified. The three specific goals of APT are presented as follows.

Goal 1 To Describe the Utilization, Technical Evolution and Cost of PT as It Enters the Mainstream

In order to optimize PT emergence, we need a means of understanding how PT therapy is being used in real time. APT would capture the clinical scenarios by disease type and stage in which PT is employed. It would also describe the demographics of PT patients (age, gender, race, and ethnicity). This utilization information would be reported in absolute terms and as a proportion of all RT patients in institutions where both PT and x-ray therapy are available and would be analyzed for changes over time. In addition, by linking into PT centers' electronic treatment management systems, the registry would also capture descriptive data summarizing variations in treatment techniques between centers. This information could be linked to publicly available Medicare reimbursement schedules to define the costs of PT treatments as a function of technique. These cost estimates could then be compared to alternative treatments.

There are other methods for capturing PT utilization, such as using claims data from insurers and billing data from providers. However, these data sources provide only high-level data by linking procedures and diagnoses. Claims and billing data would not provide sufficient details either regarding PT techniques or regarding patient characteristics. Hospital-based tumor registries and the SEER-Medicare registry link treatments to basic clinical data; however, they do not provide important technical information about the treatment technique. In addition, because these registries have a broad mission, the data are only available after a significant time lag, on the order of years for the SEER-Medicare registry. This pace of data collection would not afford the opportunity for timely studies that have the potential to trigger the emergence of PT in approximately real time.

Goal 2   To Monitor Cancer-Control and Treatment-Toxicity Outcomes for the Most Common PT Treatments

In order to impact PT emergence, we must also understand how PT outcomes vary with different treatment protocols with respect to both cancer control and toxicity. For this purpose, APT would use a cancer-outcome-surveillance system. The registry would be linked with the electronic medical records used at PT centers to capture cancer-control and acute and late radiation-toxicity outcomes as they are recorded by physicians, nurses, and patients. For the most common clinical scenarios, the registry would use a predefined set of statistical tools to determine whether a particular treatment technique or technology is associated with significantly better or worse cancer-control and toxicity outcomes. For example, late rectal bleeding is an important side effect of radiation treatments to the prostate, but an overall rate of bleeding is difficult to appreciate from the physician's perspective because rectal bleeding is delayed and episodic.[1] To monitor rectal toxicity related to PT, APT would develop a regression model that includes late rectal bleeding as the outcome and radiation modality (IMRT, double scattering PT, uniform scanning PT, or pencil-beam-scanning PT) as an explanatory variable along with other possible explanatory variables and confounders. If indeed various radiation modalities are associated with significantly different rates of rectal toxicity, this would be identified by the regression tool. Of course, this sort of outcome could be found using traditional retrospective study methods. However, via a registry, we could expect to identify these rapidly enough to influence PT techniques and technologies as centers are adopting them.

---

[1] Radiation side effects that are late and episodic are particularly difficult to appreciate from the physician's perspective without systematic data collection and analyses. Consider, for example, the side effect of late rectal bleeding, which is an effect that can occur up to 3 years after treatment but typically is self-limiting and persists less than a year. Assume that a radiation oncologist uses two different radiation techniques to treat prostate cancer—double scattering PT and pencil beam scanning PT. Assume also that there are two different radiation delivery methods and that double scattering PT is associated with a 10% risk of late rectal bleeding rate and pencil beam scanning PT, a 20% risk. Although this difference in risk is substantial and may be associated with a significant difference in the overall quality of life, the difference from the radiation oncologist's perspective would be almost imperceptible. Radiation oncologists typically follow prostate cancer patients who show no evidence of recurrence for 5 years after treatment and during that time have approximately 10 follow-up visits, once every 3 to 6 months for the first 2 years, then annually thereafter. Therefore, the radiation oncologist would see rectal bleeding associated with double scattering PT in approximately 1% to 2% of his or her prostate cancer follow-up visits, because the side effect is episodic and might only be discussed in one or two of the 10 total follow-up visits. In contrast, he or she would see rectal bleeding associated with pencil beam scanning PT in approximately 2% to 4% of his or her prostate cancer follow-up visits. Without systematic collection and comparison of toxicities, the radiation oncologist would likely perceive that the rate of late rectal bleeding is low for both double scattering and pencil beam scanning. These kinds of toxicity differences are usually discovered by the radiation oncology community through periodic retrospective reviews at academic centers. Yet, even for the largest academic centers, the time required to collect enough cases with both kinds of treatments or to coordinate a retrospective study with another institution delays these subtle but important discoveries by many years.

Goal 3   To Establish a Bioinformatics Infrastructure for Participating Centers That Allows for Shared, Prospective, Clinical, and Comparative Effectiveness Studies

APT could play an important role in the emergence of PT by facilitating PBCSs in the following two ways. First, the APT database would be a source of hypothesis-generating retrospective studies that would motivate PBCSs. The database would also provide robust baseline-outcome estimates necessary to design PBCSs. Second, it would provide a network of PT centers with informatics systems already linked through the registry. PBCS investigators could recruit centers from the networks and make use of the common clinical trial management systems already in place.

Registry Features Necessary for Achieving These Goals

In order to achieve these goals, APT would need to be adaptive, adequately representative with respect to geography and clinical setting, and inclusive of all stakeholders.

APT Must be Self-Informing and Adaptive

A registry designed to capture and monitor the most common uses of PT therapy today may be inadequate for PT therapy in a few years. Therefore, APT would need to be self-informing and adaptive. PT utilization reviews from one year should ultimately lead to research that affects PT utilization in subsequent years through the process of an adaptive registry cycle.

For example, at present, hepatocellular carcinoma (HCC) is rarely treated using radiation therapy in the United States. Therefore, APT may not initially establish a statistical surveillance system to monitor the cancer-control and toxicity outcomes of HCC. However, there are emerging data from PT centers in Japan and ongoing studies in the United States, which suggest that PT may play an important role in the management of this common malignancy (25). If future utilization reviews indicate that PT treatments for HCC are increasing, APT would then develop surveillance tools to monitor HCC outcomes. In this way, outcome reviews will be informed by utilization reviews. Furthermore, outcome reviews of HCC may suggest that one PT technique (e.g., pencil-beam scanning) is less effective than another (e.g., double scattering). Such an outcome could motivate a more detailed retrospective study using the registry database or a prospective study that could be completed using the registry bioinformatics infrastructure. Therefore, retrospective and prospective PT studies will be informed by the registry-outcome reviews. If further studies confirm that one PT technique is less effective than another, this would result in a change in the utilization of PT, which could be confirmed in subsequent utilization reviews. Multiple iterations of this cycle would optimize the emergence of PT therapy for HCC.

APT Must Include a Geographically and Clinically Diverse Set of PT Centers

Practice patterns vary geographically and by clinical setting (university practice and community practice). In order to optimize the emergence of PT, it would be important to include a diverse group of centers that adequately represent where and how PT is used.

APT Must be Representative of all Stakeholders

APT would need to evolve as PT emerges. In order to ensure that it evolves in a manner consistent with national interests, the committees that define the direction of APT need input from all stakeholders, including providers from university and community-practice settings, payers, patients, and government health care agencies.

Disease-Specific Registries of PT

The nationally representative procedure registry proposed earlier is an ambitious goal. In the meantime, single-institution or multi-institution disease-specific registries that may have more detailed outcomes and toxicity assessments could also play an important role in the emergence of PT. Indeed, Table 1 suggests that many of these are underway.

■ CONCLUSIONS

We have shown that due to the expected increase in demand for PT, clinical studies clarifying its use and efficacy are urgently needed. Although the number of clinical studies of PT is currently limited, there is a clear trend toward improved evidence development. To optimize the emergence of PT, both traditional PBCSs and patient registries will be needed.

■ ACKNOWLEDGMENTS

We would like to thank the following individuals who informed or edited this manuscript: John Cameron, Tom DeLaney, Kim Hahn, Steven Lin, Tom Merchant, Jeff Michalski, Amanda Prince, Sandra Teichman, Angela Tseng, and Barbara Winrich.

■ REFERENCES

1. www.aoa.gov/aoaroot/aging_statistics/future_growth.aspx#age. Accessed July 27, 2010.
2. www.procure.com/therapycenters. Accessed July 17, 2010.
3. Mell LK, Mehrotra AK, Mundt AJ. Intensity-modulated radiation therapy use in the U.S., 2004. *Cancer.* 2005;104(6):1296–1303.
4. Federal Register 42 CFR Part 405. Criteria for making coverage decisions. http://fdsys.gpo.gov/fdsys/pkg/FR-2000–05-16/pdf/00–12237.pdf. Accessed June 14, 2010
5. Neumann PJ, Tunis SR. Medicare and medical technology–the growing demand for relevant outcomes. *N Engl J Med.* 2010;362(5):377–379.
6. Orszag PR, Emanuel EJ. Health care reform and cost control. *N Engl J Med.* 2010;363(7):601–603.
7. Trikalinos TA, Terasawa T, Ip S, Raman G, Lau J, Tufts Medical Center Evidence-based Practice Center. *Particle Beam Radiation Therapies for Cancer. Technical Brief No. 1.* Rockville, MD: Agency for Healthcare Research and Quality. September 2009. Available at: www.effectivehealthcare.ahrq.gov/reports/final.cfm.
8. Desjardins L, Lumbroso L, Levy C, et al. [Treatment of uveal melanoma with iodine 125 plaques or proton beam therapy: indications and comparison of local recurrence rates]. *J Fr Ophtalmol.* 2003;26(3):269–276.
9. Seddon JM, Gragoudas ES, Egan KM, et al. Relative survival rates after alternative therapies for uveal melanoma. *Ophthalmology.* 1990;97(6):769–777.
10. Wilson MW, Hungerford JL. Comparison of episcleral plaque and proton beam radiation therapy for the treatment of choroidal melanoma. *Ophthalmology.* 1999;106(8):1579–1587.
11. Seddon JM, Gragoudas ES, Albert DM, Hsieh CC, Polivogianis L, Friedenberg GR. Comparison of survival rates for patients with uveal melanoma after treatment with proton beam irradiation or enucleation. *Am J Ophthalmol.* 1985;99(3):282–290.
12. Galbraith ME, Ramirez JM, Pedro LW. Quality of life, health outcomes, and identity for patients with prostate cancer in five different treatment groups. *Oncol Nurs Forum.* 2001;28(3):551–560.
13. Duttenhaver JR, Shipley WU, Perrone T, et al. Protons or megavoltage X-rays as boost therapy for patients irradiated for localized prostatic carcinoma. An early phase I/II comparison. *Cancer.* 1983;51(9):1599–1604.
14. Shipley WU, Verhey LJ, Munzenrider JE, et al. Advanced prostate cancer: the results of a randomized comparative trial of high dose irradiation boosting with conformal protons compared with conventional dose irradiation using photons alone. *Int J Radiat Oncol Biol Phys.* 1995;32(1):3–12.
15. Guidelines for the use of proton radiation therapy in National Cancer Institute sponsored cooperative group clinical trials. www3.cancer.gov/rrp/proton.doc. Accessed July 15, 2010.
16. Brada M, Pijls-Johannesma M, De Ruysscher D. Proton therapy in clinical practice: current clinical evidence. *J Clin Oncol.* 2007;25(8):965–970.
17. Goitein M, Cox JD. Should randomized clinical trials be required for proton radiotherapy? *J Clin Oncol.* 2008;26(2):175–176.
18. Brada M, De Ruysscher D, Pijls-Johannesma M. Evidence for proton therapy. *J Clin Oncol.* 2008;26(15):2592–2593.

19. Teppe JE. Protons and parachutes. *J Clin Oncol.* 2008; 26(15):2436–2437.

20. Glatstein E, Glick J, Kaiser L, Hahn SM. Should randomized clinical trials be required for proton radiotherapy? An alternative view. *J Clin Oncol.* 2008; 26(15):2438–2439.

21. Packer RJ, Goldwein J, Nicholson HS, et al. Treatment of children with medulloblastomas with reduced-dose craniospinal radiation therapy and adjuvant chemotherapy: a Children's Cancer Group Study. *J Clin Oncol.* 1999;17(7):2127–2136.

22. Fossati P, Ricardi U, Orecchia R. Pediatric medulloblastoma: toxicity of current treatment and potential role of protontherapy. *Cancer Treat Rev.* 2009; 35(1):79–96.

23. Pijls-Johannesma M, Grutters JP, Verhaegen F, Lambin P, De Ruysscher D. Do we have enough evidence to implement particle therapy as standard treatment in lung cancer? A systematic literature review. *Oncologist.* 2010;15(1):93–103.

24. Gliklich RE, Dreyer NA, eds. *Registries for Evaluating Patient Outcomes: A User's Guide.* (Prepared by Outcome DEcIDE Center [Outcome Sciences, Inc. dba Outcome] under Contract No. HHSA29020050035ITO1.) AHRQ Publication No. 07-EHC001–1. Rockville, MD: Agency for Healthcare Research and Quality. April 2007.

25. Fukumitsu N, Sugahara S, Nakayama H, et al. A prospective study of hypofractionated proton beam therapy for patients with hepatocellular carcinoma. *Int J Radiat Oncol Biol Phys.* 2009;74(3):831–836.

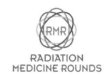

RADIATION
MEDICINE ROUNDS

Review of Proton-Beam Radiotherapy of Prostate Cancer

Carl J. Rossi, Jr.*

Loma Linda University Medical Center, Loma Linda, CA

■ ABSTRACT

Proton-beam-radiation therapy of organ-confined prostate cancer now constitutes one of the most commonly treated malignancies with this modality. Because of this, questions have been raised regarding the efficacy and cost-effectiveness of such treatment. This chapter briefly discusses the history of proton-beam-radiation therapy, details the clinical results obtained with proton therapy to date, reviews ongoing clinical trials, and seeks to place proton-beam therapy in the context of other technological evolutions in radiation oncology.

Keywords: protons, prostate cancer, dose escalation

■ INTRODUCTION

Prostate cancer presents a major oncologic dilemma for the developed world. In the United States there will be an estimated 192,280 new cases diagnosed in 2009, with approximately 27,000 deaths from this disease (1). Prostate cancer is the second leading cause of cancer deaths among American men and accounts for approximately 10% of all cancer-related deaths in men. A similar incidence and death rate is seen in Western Europe, with the lowest reported incidence being in Eastern/Southern Asia. Over the past 20 years, the discovery and use of prostate-specific antigen (PSA) as a screening tool has led to both an increase in the number of cases being diagnosed and a decrease in the proportion of men being diagnosed with advanced disease. This trend toward diagnosis with organ-confined disease has prompted the development and refinement of treatment methods directed at the prostate in the entirely reasonable hope of providing long-term disease-free survival and cure.

From the standpoint of radiotherapy, virtually all technical advances in prostate cancer treatment have primarily been implemented to reduce normal

*Corresponding author, Department of Radiation Medicine, Loma Linda University Medical Center, 11234 Anderson St., Room B-124, Loma Linda CA, 92354
E-mail address: crossi@llurm.org

Radiation Medicine Rounds 1:3 (2010) 471–490.
DOI: 10.5003/2151–4208.1.3.471

tissue toxicity by limiting the volume of adjacent bladder and rectum that receive high doses of radiation. A direct consequence of this improvement in dose conformality has been dose escalation (2–7), a concept whose clinical utility has been tested and confirmed in one proton-beam-based prospective, randomized phase III trial.

The unique physical properties inherent in proton beams makes them particularly attractive to the radiation oncologist, for they permit a reduction in "integral dose" (defined as the total radiation dose given to the patient) over and above anything that can be achieved with photon-based external beam treatment systems (8–12).

However, proton-beam therapy of prostate cancer is not without its detractors. Critics often point out that a multitude of effective treatment methods exist and that modern photon therapy using intensity-modulated techniques (IMRT) and image-guided treatment delivery (IGRT) yield similar outcomes at less monetary cost to society, and still others question the wisdom of aggressively treating prostate cancer at all (13,14). These criticisms force one to ask the question: Is prostate cancer a good candidate for proton-beam therapy? Answering this question will first depend on a review of the available data demonstrating the clinical utility of proton-beam therapy in the treatment of prostate cancer and the future potentials inherent in this modality.

■ EARLY PROTON-BEAM TREATMENT RESULTS

The ability to use proton-beam therapy to treat deep organs was, and is, greatly dependent on the concurrent ongoing development of cross-sectional imaging technology (CT, MRI) and modern computers; hence, it is not surprising that proton-beam therapy of prostate cancer did not commence until the late 1970s. Beginning in 1977, Shipley and associates at the Massachusetts General Hospital (MGH) initiated a phase I trial in which proton-beam radiotherapy

was used to give a boost dose to patients with locally advanced disease who were also receiving photon radiotherapy. At that time, this boost dose was felt to be over and above what could be safely given with existing photon technology. Seventeen patients with stage T2 to T4 disease received a perineally directed proton-beam boost of 20 to 26 Gy (given at a rate of 1.8–2 Gy/day) following treatment to the prostate and pelvis to a dose of 50.4 Gy with 10-MV photons. A perineal approach was chosen because this was the only anatomical pathway that allowed the 160-MeV proton beam generated by the Harvard Cyclotron to reliably encompass the entire prostate gland. Acutely, the treatment was well tolerated and after a follow-up period ranging from 12 to 27 months no severe late rectal reactions were noted (15).

■ HARVARD RANDOMIZED TRIAL

These favorable toxicity results led directly to the initiation of a prospective, randomized trial designed to test the benefits of proton-beam dose escalation in patients with locally advanced disease. Patients with stage T3 to T4 tumors were chosen as it was felt that this group stood to gain the most benefit from high doses. All patients received 50.4 Gy to the prostate and pelvis with megavoltage photons. They were then randomized to receive either an additional 16.8 Gy of photons (for a total prostate dose of 67.2 Gy) or 25.2 GyE of protons for a total prostate dose of 75.6 Gy. Adjuvant hormonal therapy was not permitted. The limited availability of the Harvard Cyclotron affected patient accrual; nonetheless, 202 patients were eventually enrolled, with 103 of them being treated in the high-dose arm and 99 in the standard-dose arm.

With a median follow-up of 61 months, there were no differences seen in overall survival, disease-specific survival, total relapse-free survival, or local control between the arms. Patients with high-grade tumors who were treated on the high-dose arm did experience an improvement in local control at 5 and 8 years (92% and 77% vs. 80% and 60%, P = .89). Patients whose digital rectal exams normalized following treatment and who underwent subsequent prostate biopsy revealed a lower positive biopsy rate in the high-dose arm (28% vs. 45%), and, perhaps most surprisingly, the local control rates for patients with Gleason grade 4 to 5 tumors (57 patients total) were significantly better at 5 and 8 years in the high-dose patients (94% and 84% vs. 68% and 19%, P = 0.001). High-dose treatment was associated with an increase in late grade 1 to 2 rectal bleeding (32% vs. 12%, P = 0.02) (16).

These results have been erroneously cited by some as evidence that proton-beam dose escalation is of doubtful utility (17). It should be noted that the patients treated in this trial were at a high risk of not only local failure but of distant failure; therefore, one should not be surprised that overall survival was unaffected by a purely local treatment intervention. In addition, patients with these adverse characteristics would not, if diagnosed today, receive radiotherapy as monotherapy and instead would be treated with a multimodality approach (18–22). The two most important facts learned from this study are (a) high-dose radiotherapy did decrease local failure, and this decrease was most profound in those patients with the most aggressive tumors, and (b) dose escalation by means of a perineal proton beam (an approach that has largely been abandoned today as higher-energy machines have become available) can be performed safely with acceptable toxicity (23).

The improvement in local control seen with dose escalation prompted a very logical question: If patients with earlier-stage disease who are less likely to have already experienced metastatic failure are treated with dose escalation, will we see a positive effect on survival? This intriguing hypothesis has been tested in a prospective, randomized multi-institution trial, and its conclusions will be covered, presently.

■ LOMA LINDA UNIVERSITY MEDICAL CENTER-INITIAL EXPERIENCE

The completion in 1990 of the world's first hospital-based proton treatment center at Loma Linda University Medical Center (LLUMC) marked the beginning of a transition in proton-beam therapy from the research laboratory setting to that of clinical radiation oncology (24). Beginning in late 1991, prostate patients at LLUMC were treated on a clinical trial that set out to confirm the efficacy and toxicity data generated at MGH. Between December 1991 and December 1995, a total of 643 patients were treated to total prostate radiation doses of 74 to 75 GyE. Patients who were deemed to be at a low risk for occult nodal metastasis were treated with lateral proton beams alone, whereas those who were felt to benefit from elective nodal radiation received 45 Gy to the pelvis with 18- to 23-MV photons delivered via a multifield three-dimensional conformal technique. Patient characteristics are shown in Table 1.

TABLE 1

Pretreatment characteristics of prostate cancer patients treated at Loma Linda University Medical Center

		No. of Patients
Stage	1A/1B	28
	1C	91
	2A	157
	2B	173
	2C	157
	3	37
Gleason	2–5	232
	6–7	324
	8–10	54
Initial PSA	≤4.0	53
	4.1–10.0	280
	10.0–20.0	175
	>20.0	85

From Ref. 25.

With a median follow-up of 43 months, the overall biochemical disease-free survival (bNED) rate was 79% as per the American Society for Therapeutic Radiology and Oncology (ASTRO) definition of three successively rising PSA values above a nadir equating to biochemical failure. The risk of biochemical failure was strongly dependent on the pretreatment PSA with 5-year bNED survival rates varying from 53% in patients with pretreatment PSAs of 20% to 50%, and even up to 100%, with PSAs < 4.1 (Figure 1). bNED survival was also significantly influenced by posttreatment PSA nadir. A multivariant analysis of failure predictors demonstrated that initial stage, PSA, and Gleason Score were all strong predictors of biochemical failure at 5 years (Table 2). As was also reported in the MGH trial, treatment was by and large well tolerated. Acute toxicity was minimal, and all patients completed the prescribed course of radiotherapy. Proctitis remained the most common late toxicity with grade 2 toxicity occurring in 21% of patients at 3 years; for the majority of patients this represented a single episode of rectal bleeding. No ≥ grade 3 gastrointestinal (GI)

toxicity was seen. Grade 2 genitourinary (GU) toxicity (primarily gross hematuria) was seen in 5.4% of patients at 3 years, with two patients developing grade 3 bladder toxicity. Interestingly, no significant difference in late toxicity was seen between those patients treated with protons alone and those receiving pelvic x-ray therapy. The excellent biochemical control rates and acceptable toxicity seen in this trial confirmed the earlier MGH data and led to the implementation of a prospective, randomized dose-escalation study in organ-confined prostate cancer (25).

A further update of the initial LLUMC experience was published in 2004. This study encompassed 1,255 patients with stage T1 to T3 disease who were treated with proton-beam radiotherapy alone (i.e., no prior or concurrent hormonal therapy) to a dose of 74 to 75 GyE. As was seen in the earlier trial, initial PSA, Gleason Grade, and PSA nadir were all strong predictors of bNED survival (Figures 2–4). Treatment continued to be well tolerated with rates of Radiation Therapy Oncology Group (RTOG) grade ≥ 3 GI/GU late morbidity of <1% (26).

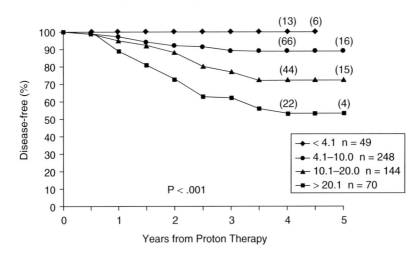

FIGURE 1
Risk of subsequent biochemical failure versus initial PSA in patients treated at Loma Linda University Medical Center (25).

TABLE 2
Multivariate analysis of failure predictors in patients treated at Loma Linda University Medical Center[a]

		% Disease-Free Survival 5 Years	Univariate P	Multivariate P
Initial PSA	≤4.0	100		
	4.1–10.0	88	<0.001	0.001
	10.0–20.0	68		
	>20.0	48		
Gleason	2–5	82		
	6–7	76	<0.001	0.007
	8–10	48		
T stage	1A/1B	79		
	1C	94		
	2A	87	<0.001	0.003
	2B	73		
	2C	59		
	3	59		

[a] From Ref. 25.

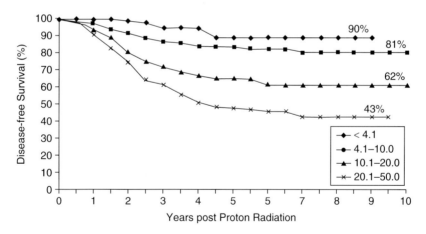

FIGURE 2
Initial PSA versus biochemical survival-updated Loma Linda data (26).

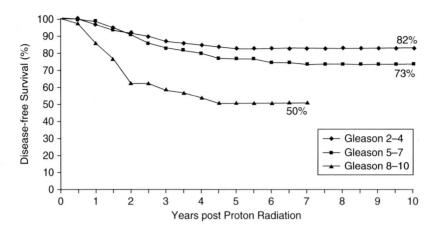

FIGURE 3
Gleason score versus biochemical survival-updated Loma Linda data (26).

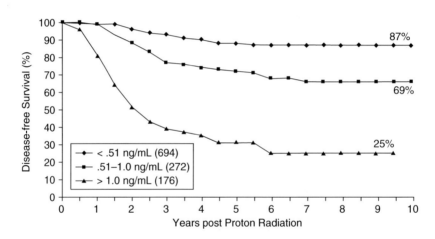

FIGURE 4
PSA Nadir versus biochemical survival-updated Loma Linda data (26).

■ PROTON RADIATION ONCOLOGY GROUP PROSPECTIVE, RANDOMIZED TRIAL

Beginning in 1996, LLUMC and MGH embarked on the Proton Radiation Oncology Group/American College of Radiology (PROG/ACR) 95–09 trial, a prospective, randomized dose-escalation study for patients with organ-confined prostate cancer. This study was designed to test the hypothesis that a dose escalation from 70.2 to 79.2 GyE would result in a statistically significant decrease in local failure, biochemical failure, and overall survival. Eligibility criteria included stage T1b to T2b disease (as per the 1992 American Joint Committee on Cancer staging system), a PSA of

≤15 ng/mL, and no evidence of metastatic disease on imaging studies (bone scan, abdomino-pelvic CT scan). Gleason score was not an exclusion criterion, and no prior or concurrent androgen-deprivation therapy was permitted. Pretreatment patient characteristics are shown in Table 3.

Patients were randomly assigned to receive a total prostate dose of 70.2 or 79.2 GyE. Radiotherapy was administered sequentially in two phases. In phase I, conformal proton beams were used to treat the prostate alone. Depending on randomization either 19.8 or 28.8 GyE in 11 or 16 fractions was delivered. The clinical target volume (CTV) was the prostate with a 5-mm margin. Beam arrangement was facility dependent with patients at LLUMC being treated with lateral proton beams of 225- to 250-MeV energy, whereas at MGH a perineal 160-MeV proton beam was employed. Before each proton-beam treatment a water balloon was inserted into the rectum and inflated with 50 to 100 mL of saline; this served the dual purpose of distending the rectal lumen to decrease the integral dose to the rectum and minimizing prostate motion.

In the second phase of treatment, all patients received 50.4 Gy of photons given in 1.8 Gy fractions. The CTV was the prostate and seminal vesicles. No effort was made to include the pelvic lymphatics. Three-dimensional planning was used on all patients, and photon energies of 10 to 23 MV were used. The use of photons for a portion of the treatment was solely to allow both institutions to participate in this trial, for at the time the trial commenced MGH patients were still restricted to treatment at the Harvard Cyclotron Laboratory and the limited throughput of that facility meant that the most efficient use of protons was as a boost and not as monotherapy. The randomization schema is shown in Figure 5. A total of 393 patients were randomized between January 1996 and December 1999.

The results of the trial were initially published in 2005 (27), with an update in 2010. At a median follow-up of 8.9 years there is a persistent and statistically significant increase in biochemical freedom from relapse among patients randomized to the high-dose arm (Figure 6). This difference was seen when using both the ASTRO and the more recent Phoenix definition (28) (in which biochemical failure = a PSA elevation of > 2 ng/mL above a nadir). Subgroup analysis showed a particularly strong benefit in 10-year bNED survival among the "low-risk" patients (defined as PSA < 10 ng/mL, and Gleason score < 7 and stage < t2b), with 92.2% of high-dose patients being disease free versus 78.8% for standard dose (P = .0001). A strong trend toward a similar positive finding was seen in the intermediate risk patients, but this has not yet reached statistical significance (Figure 7). In addition, patients in the standard-dose arm are twice as likely to have been started on androgen deprivation therapy as high-dose patients (22 vs. 11, P = 0.47) with such treatment usually being initiated due to a rising PSA. To date, there is no difference in overall survival between the arms (29).

As was seen in the previously reported proton trials treatment was well tolerated. Only 2% of patients in both arms have experienced late GU toxicities of grade ≥ 3 and 1% have experienced late GI toxicity of grade ≥ 3. Interestingly, as opposed to what has been reported in some photon-based, randomized dose-escalation trials, high-dose radiotherapy delivered via a conformal proton-beam boost did not result in an increase in late grade ≥ 3 GI morbidity among the high-dose patients (Table 4). This encouraging finding has been confirmed by a patient-reported sensitive Quality Of Life instrument that did not report any greater late morbidity than the physician-reported scores, and which revealed equal and high satisfaction with quality of life between both arms (30).

Thus, the PROG/ACR 9509 trial provides "level 1" evidence verifying the importance of radiation dose escalation in organ-confined prostate cancer, and, although this study was not designed to directly compare the efficacy of conformal proton-beam radiotherapy against other conformal techniques or modalities, it does

TABLE 3

Pretreatment patient characteristics of prostate cancer patients treated on the PROG/ACR 9509 prospective randomized phase III dose-escalation study[a]

| Characteristic | Assigned Dose | | | |
| | 70.2 GyE (n = 196) | | 79.2 GyE (n = 195) | |
	No.	%	No.	%
Age (y)				
45–59	43	22	34	17
60–69	92	47	106	54
70–79	61	31	55	28
≥80	1	0.5	0	
Median	67		66	
Range	45–91		47–78	
Race				
White	175	89	178	91
Hispanic	4	2	7	3
Black	12	6	5	3
Other	5	3	5	3
PSA (ng/mL)				
<5	54	28	47	24
5 to <10	114	58	119	61
10–15	28	14	29	15
Median	6.3		6.2	
Range	1.24–14.68		0.67–14.30	
Kamfosky performance status				
80	8	4	9	5
90	52	27	47	24
100	136	69	139	71
Combined Gleason				
2–6	148	75	147	75
7	29	15	30	15
8–10	18	9	15	8
Unknown	1	1	3	2
T stage				
T1b	1	1	0	
T1c	120	61	120	61
T2a	43	22	50	26
T2b	32	16	25	13
N stage				
N0	0		2	1
NX	196	100	193	99
Risk groups*				
Low	111	57	116	59
Intermediate	75	38	69	35
High	10	5	7	4
Not classified	0		3	2

Abbreviations: GyE, gray equivalents; PSA, prostate-specific antigen.

[a] From Ref. 27.

* Risk groups according to D'Amico et al. (23).

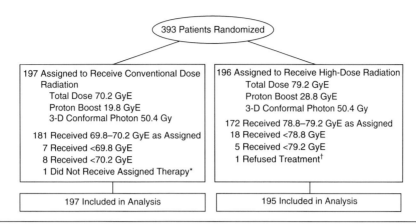

FIGURE 5
Patient randomization schemata for the PROG/ACR 9509 Trial (27).

demonstrate that conformal proton-beam radiotherapy is an effective treatment for this disease, with minimal risk of experiencing severe treatment-induced toxicity.

■ UNIVERSITY OF FLORIDA

The University of Florida Proton Therapy Institute opened in the summer of 2006 with prostate cancer treatment commencing at that time. From August 2006 to October 2007, 211 patients were treated on one of three prospective trials: 78 GyE/39 fractions for low-risk disease, dose escalation from 78 to 82 GyE for intermediate-risk disease, and 78 GyE with concomitant taxotere, followed by androgen-deprivation therapy, for high-risk disease. Preliminary GI and GU toxicity data were reported in 2009 with a minimum of 1-year follow-up. At end of 6 months into the follow-up period, there were 47 grade 2 toxicities and one

grade 3 GU toxicity, and, at 12 months, there were 48 grade 2 toxicities and one grade 3 toxicity. The overwhelming majority of grade 2 symptoms (98%) were retentive symptoms requiring treatment with α-blockers. Multivariate analysis suggested that grade 2+ GU toxicities were correlated with pretreatment prostatitis, pretreatment International Prostate Symptom Score (IPSS) score, and, as time progressed, with patient age and pretreatment GU symptom management. This strongly suggests that the predominant predictors of early GU toxicity were pretreatment clinical factors.

GI toxicities were considerably less common, with one grade 2 and no grade 3 or greater toxicities at 6 months, increasing to eight grade 2 toxicities and just one grade 3 toxicity at 12 months. Two grade 2 toxicities occurred on both the low-risk and high-risk protocol, and the remainder occurred on the dose-escalation intermediate-risk study. Univariate analysis of the low- and intermediate-risk patients revealed a significant

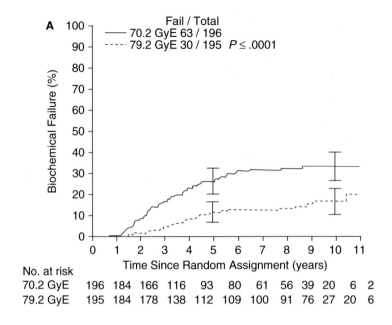

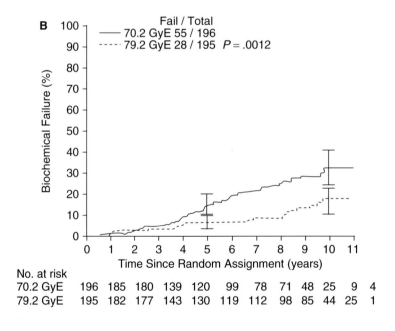

FIGURE 6

Biochemical freedom from relapse versus prostate radiation dose. (A) Biochemical failure by ASTRO consensus. (B) Biochemical failure by Phoenix criteria. Updated data from the PROG/ACR 9509 phase III trial (29).

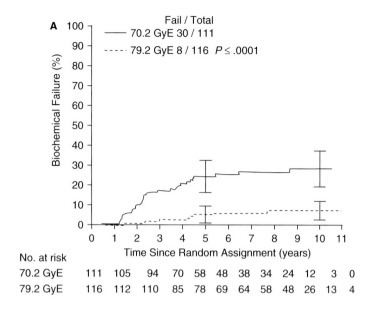

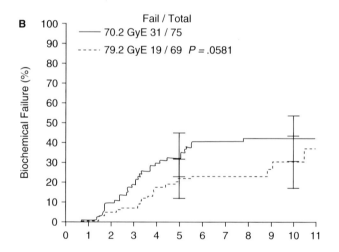

FIGURE 7
Biochemical failure by American Society for Therapeutic Radiology and Oncology Consensus definition after conventional and high-dose conformal radiotherapy. (A) Biochemical failure for the low-risk group. (B) Biochemical failure for the intermediate risk group. Abbreviation: GyE, gray equivalent (29).

TABLE 6
Acute GI/GU morbidities at the Hyogo Ion Beam Medical Center[a]

Toxicity	Grade 0	Grade 1	Grade 2	Grade 3	Grade 4
Dysuria	52 (18)	134 (47)	101 (35)	0	0
Urinary frequency	69 (24)	179 (62)	36 (13)	3 (1)	0
Urinary retention	204 (71)	73 (25	9 (3)	1 (0.3)	0
Hematuria	231 (81)	50 (17)	5 (2)	1 (0.3)	0
GU, overall	18 (6)	154 (54)	111 (39)	4 (1)	0
Proctitis	282 (98)	5 (2)	0	0	0
Rectal bleeding	0	0	0	0	0
GI, overall	282 (98)	5 (2)	0	0	0

Abbreviations: GU, genitourinary; GI, gastrointestinal; NCI-CTC, National Cancer Institute Common Toxicity Criteria.

[a] From Ref. 33.

Data presented as number of patients, with percentages in parentheses.

late bladder/rectal toxicity. This difference in α/β ratios implies that prostate cancer cells are more sensitive to changes in radiation fraction size than the bladder and the rectum are, meaning that, by increasing the daily fraction size and reducing the total radiation dose, one can potentially shorten the overall treatment time without compromising tumor control and without increasing the risk of incurring a late GI/GU injury.

Hypofractionation has a long-established history in proton-beam therapy and is now routinely employed in proton-beam treatment of ocular melanomas (35–37), intracranial metastasis, arterial-venous malformations (38,39), lung cancer (40), and breast cancer (41). It also is being actively investigated in prostate cancer, although to date this investigation has employed primarily IMRT-based approaches (42–46). There is an emerging body of data supporting its safety and efficacy in this setting to the point that at least one prominent radiation biologist has declared that hypofractionation should be considered the treatment of choice for prostate cancer (47).

At the time of this writing, there are two hypofractionated conformal proton-beam treatment protocols actively accruing patients in the United States.

At LLUMC, a phase I to phase II trial of 60 GyE/20 fractions (which is designed to be isoeffective with 81 GyE/ 45 fractions assuming an α/β ratio of 1.5 for prostate cancer) began accruing patients in 2009. Eligibility is limited to "low-risk" patients (PSA < 10 ng/mL, Gleason < 7, and Stage < T2b). Preliminary analysis indicates that treatment is well tolerated with no patient (n = 50) experiencing a grade ≥ 3 acute GI/GU complication. Posttreatment PSA decreases are consistent with expectations. At the University of Florida hypofractionation is being investigated in a similar protocol in which patients with low- to intermediate-risk prostate cancer are treated on a 5-week hypofractionated regimen to a total dose of 70 GyE/28 fractions for low-risk patients and 72.5 GyE/29 fractions for intermediate risk patients.

■ PROTON-BEAM RADIOTHERAPY OF PROSTATE CANCER-SUMMARY

The published peer-reviewed data conclusively demonstrate that conformal proton-beam radiotherapy is extremely well tolerated and that it can reliably produce bNED survival rates equivalent to other modern radiotherapy modalities and to radical prostatectomy. Conformal proton-beam dose escalation has been tested in a prospective, randomized trial and has been shown to improve bNED survival without (as opposed to what has been seen in some IMRT trials (48)) concurrently increasing the risk of late grade ≥ 3 GI/GU morbidity. However, attempts to escalate dose to 82 GyE have been met with a substantial increase in late GI morbidity; this may reflect the "limit" beyond which treatment with passive-scattered beams and their attendant substantial penumbra may not be safely possible, although it is likely that the pending introduction of intensity-modulated proton therapy (IMPT) via active beam scanning and the implementation of novel image-guided techniques will permit further increases in dose. Hypofractionation is currently being tested in protocols at several proton centers, and preliminary data on the safety and efficacy of this technique will be available within the next 12 to 18 months.

■ THE FUTURE OF PROTON-BEAM RADIOTHERAPY OF PROSTATE CANCER—PITFALLS AND POSSIBILITIES

Now that we have reviewed the available data on proton-beam therapy, it is time to return to the question asked in the introduction: Is prostate cancer a good candidate for proton-beam therapy? I believe that the evidence-based answer has to be an unqualified "yes." The rationale supporting this conclusion is found in the data. Treatment-related morbidity is low, whereas biochemical freedom from relapse is equivalent to other radiotherapy techniques. The PROG/ACR 9509 trial provides "level 1" evidence strongly supporting the benefits of dose escalation in organ-confined prostate cancer. Furthermore, it demonstrated that when conformal proton beams are used to escalate the dose, this dose escalation can be achieved without increasing the risk of incurring moderate to severe treatment-related morbidity, something that has not always been the case with IMRT-derived dose escalation. In addition, these results are repeatable,

as evidenced by the minimal morbidity reported in the several thousand prostate patients treated at multiple proton-beam facilities worldwide.

Prostate cancer is an excellent site in which to test and perfect the implementation of new treatment techniques and dose-fractionation schedules. Ongoing technical advances in proton-beam therapy will lead to further dose specificity within the target organ and a further reduction in normal tissue radiation dose. Development of these techniques, including IMPT and real-time particle beam IGRT, will require their testing in a large number of patients who have similar disease characteristics and anatomic constraints. Prostate cancer represents an excellent "test bed" for these important developments. It is an extremely common disease, so large numbers of potential patients exist, and, as opposed to some other common tumors (most notably lung cancer), it is typically diagnosed while confined to its organ of origin so that treated patients are likely to live for many years; therefore, performing a complete analysis of late effects during the posttreatment phase is required. Organ motion is minimal, which aids in the development of beam-scanning techniques that are inherently more sensitive to target motion than are passive-scattered arrangements. Perfecting spot-scanning treatment in a system with minimal organ motion before moving on to highly mobile tumors makes a great deal more sense to me than the converse. The fact that tumor response can be assessed biochemically as opposed to clinically or radiologically means that the effects of alterations in treatment techniques on tumor can be assessed (and potentially adjusted or even abandoned) far more rapidly than when less exacting measures are available. Last, in contrast to other sites like the base of skull, the prostate is adjacent to only two critical organs about which a good deal is already known concerning dose-volume effects and their impact on acute and late morbidity, thereby providing for a more accurate extrapolation of the effects of any potential treatment alterations than would be true of other, less frequently treated sites.

One of the often-voiced complaints about proton-beam treatment is the cost of providing this therapy. This concern is commonly raised whenever any new treatment technology or, for that matter, any new technology, is introduced into society. In the health care arena, new technology is increasingly being met with the demand that the new method be subjected to randomized trials versus existing treatment methods before the new method is accepted by the medical community and health care payers. Even though at first examination this argument seems to have a certain intellectual appeal, I believe that in the case of proton-beam treatment such trials are not necessary and may even turn out to be unethical.

This clamor for randomized data is not new, nor is it confined to the introduction of proton-beam treatment. Dr. Herman Suit reminds us that similar arguments were made in the early 1960s questioning the introduction of Cobalt 60 teletherapy units into radiation oncology, arguments that, at this juncture, seem to verge upon the ridiculous (would any of us care to willingly return to the days of Orthovoltage treatment?) but were quite popular in their time (49).

In his 2001 Gray Lecture Dr. Suit goes on to state the following "four truisms" of radiation oncology (50):

- *No* advantage to *any* patient of *any* irradiation of *any* normal tissue exists.
- Direct radiation complications *never* occur in unirradiated tissues.
- That a smaller treatment volume is superior is *not* a medical research question.
- One may only investigate the magnitude of the gain or the cost of achieving that gain.

It must also be noted that virtually all other advancements in radiotherapy treatment technology, including the widespread embracement of IMRT, have not occurred only after this technology was first tested in prospective trials but only because the new technology more closely conformed to these truisms than its predecessor did. When considered

from this perspective, proton-beam therapy is correctly viewed as a further large step along the same road of technological advancement that has been followed diligently by radiation oncologists since the inception of our specialty. Considering the relative biological equivalence of protons and x-rays, and that at this juncture roughly the same total radiation dose can be given to the prostate with either technology, from a moral and practical standpoint it would be difficult, if not impossible, to compel patients to participate in a trial in which the only difference is not the expected outcome in terms of disease control but the volume of normal tissue that will be irradiated.

The monetary cost of proton-beam radiotherapy compared to other radiotherapy modalities has been an area of great interest and debate. In a widely reported 2007 analysis, Konski and associates used a mathematical model to calculate the "cost-effectiveness" of proton-beam treatment versus IMRT in organ-confined prostate cancer (13). This analysis was predicated on the assumption that proton-beam treatment would safely permit dose escalation to 91.8 GyE as opposed to 81 GyE delivered via IMRT and the impact that this dose escalation would have on a number of factors, including survival. The authors concluded that the potential benefits accrued by proton-beam therapy exceeded the "commonly accepted standard" of US$50,000/quality-adjusted-life-years (QALY) and, therefore, that it was not a cost-effective therapy.

This conclusion is founded on the assumption that the cost of proton-beam treatment will remain higher than IMRT for the foreseeable future, and the authors admit that "There is research investigating more economical methods of producing protons." This assumption will hold true only if proton-beam treatment technology, unlike the overwhelming majority of technological developments, be it in medicine or virtually all other fields of human endeavor, will not become less expensive as it becomes more widely available. Computer technology is an obvious example of this well-known principle, but ample parallels also exist in radiation oncology. Our current proton treatment centers are the technological equivalents of the 1930s Van De Graff generator-based megavoltage photon units. These were multiton, multistory behemoths that were essentially hand-built. They were so expensive, large, and complex that few hospitals could afford them, and their use was, therefore, extremely limited. This did nothing to decrease the clinical appeal of their megavoltage beams, and 80 years later their miniaturized descendants can be found throughout the developed world. Proton-beam treatment units are already experiencing the same technological development, and a number of new machine designs, ranging from compact superconducting cyclotrons to small linear accelerators, are currently in advanced stages of development. Once these units, with their lower acquisition costs, are operational the cost of proton-beam therapy will decrease accordingly, and when the cost of proton-beam treatment approximates that of IMRT, all of the current arguments over relative efficacy will in all likelihood come to an abrupt end (a position that has been most eloquently elucidated by Dr. Herman Suit). In order for proton-beam treatment to achieve this goal it has to be used for treatment of common cancers like prostate cancer. Again, this pathway is not new, and it simply mirrors the trail already blazed by other radiotherapy technologies, including IMRT.

The one area of particle-beam-based prostate cancer treatment in which I believe a randomized trial makes sense would be in a comparison of modern proton-beam treatment with heavy ion therapy. The emergence of dual proton–carbon ion centers will allow us to test in a clinical setting whether or not there is a clinical advantage to the use of high relative biological effectiveness radiation. Unlike the proton–IMRT situation, the possession of a Bragg Peak by both particles means that there is not a substantial difference in normal tissue radiation exposure between the two modalities and thus the ethical concerns over irradiating large volumes of normal tissue will no longer apply.

The prostate represents perhaps the ideal proving ground for proton-beam treatment. Rather than discourage its use on prostate cancer I believe that its use should be encouraged. The techniques perfected and lessons learned will serve to benefit all patients, including those treated with other radiotherapy modalities, and will add invaluable data to the widespread clinical implementation of proton-beam radiotherapy.

■ REFERENCES

1. NCCN Clinical Practice Guidelines in Oncology-Prostate Cancer. 2010.
2. Bergström P, Löfroth PO, Widmark A. High-precision conformal radiotherapy (HPCRT) of prostate cancer–a new technique for exact positioning of the prostate at the time of treatment. *Int J Radiat Oncol Biol Phys.* 1998;42(2):305–311.
3. Bey P, Carrie C, Beckendorf V, et al. Dose escalation with 3D-CRT in prostate cancer: French study of dose escalation with conformal 3D radiotherapy in prostate cancer-preliminary results. *Int J Radiat Oncol Biol Phys.* 2000;48(2):513–517.
4. Bolla M. What is the role of radiation dose escalation in the treatment of localized prostate cancer? *Nat Clin Pract Urol.* 2008;5(8):418–419.
5. Cheung R, Tucker SL, Dong L, Kuban D. Dose-response for biochemical control among high-risk prostate cancer patients after external beam radiotherapy. *Int J Radiat Oncol Biol Phys.* 2003;56(5):1234–1240.
6. Goldner G, Dimopoulos J, Kirisits C, Pötter R. Moderate dose escalation in three-dimensional conformal localized prostate cancer radiotherapy: single-institutional experience in 398 patients comparing 66 Gy versus 70 Gy versus 74 Gy. *Strahlenther Onkol.* 2009;185(7):438–445.
7. Zelefsky MJ, Yamada Y, Fuks Z, et al. Long-term results of conformal radiotherapy for prostate cancer: impact of dose escalation on biochemical tumor control and distant metastases-free survival outcomes. *Int J Radiat Oncol Biol Phys.* 2008;71(4):1028–1033.
8. Archambeau JO, Bennett GW, Chen ST. Potential of proton beams for total nodal irradiation. *Acta Radiol Ther Phys Biol.* 1974;13(5):393–401.
9. Arjomandy B, Sahoo N, Cox J, Lee A, Gillin M. Comparison of surface doses from spot scanning and passively scattered proton therapy beams. *Phys Med Biol.* 2009;54(14):N295–N302.

10. Loeffler JS, Smith AR, Suit HD. The potential role of proton beams in radiation oncology. *Semin Oncol.* 1997;24(6):686–695.

11. Suit H, Urie M. Proton beams in radiation therapy. *J Natl Cancer Inst.* 1992;84(3):155–164.

12. Amaldi U. Conformal radiation therapy with hadron beams and the programs of the TERA Foundation. *Rays.* 1998;23(3):486–507.

13. Konski A, Speier W, Hanlon A, Beck JR, Pollack A. Is proton beam therapy cost effective in the treatment of adenocarcinoma of the prostate? *J Clin Oncol.* 2007;25(24):3603–3608.

14. Steinberg ML, Konski A. Proton beam therapy and the convoluted pathway to incorporating emerging technology into routine medical care in the United States. *Cancer J.* 2009;15(4):333–338.

15. Shipley WU, Tepper JE, Prout GR Jr, et al. Proton radiation as boost therapy for localized prostatic carcinoma. *JAMA.* 1979;241(18):1912–1915.

16. Shipley WU, Verhey LJ, Munzenrider JE, et al. Advanced prostate cancer: the results of a randomized comparative trial of high dose irradiation boosting with conformal protons compared with conventional dose irradiation using photons alone. *Int J Radiat Oncol Biol Phys.* 1995;32(1):3–12.

17. Hanks GE. A question-filled future for dose escalation in prostate cancer. *Int J Radiat Oncol Biol Phys.* 1995;32(1):267–269.

18. Wiegel T, Hinkelbein W. [Locally advanced prostate carcinoma (T2b-T4 N0) without and with clinical evidence of local progression (Tx N+) with lymphatic metastasis. Is radiotherapy for pelvic lymphatic metastasis indicated or not?]. *Strahlenther Onkol.* 1998;174(5):231–236.

19. Roach M 3rd. Neoadjuvant total androgen suppression and radiotherapy in the management of locally advanced prostate cancer. *Semin Urol Oncol.* 1996;14(2 suppl 2):32–7; discussion 38.

20. Roach M 3rd. Neoadjuvant therapy prior to radiotherapy for clinically localized prostate cancer. *Eur Urol.* 1997;32(suppl 3):48–54.

21. Roach M 3rd. Current status of androgen suppression and radiotherapy for patients with prostate cancer. *J Steroid Biochem Mol Biol.* 1999;69(1–6):239–245.

22. Roach M. Neoadjuvant hormonal therapy in men being treated with radiotherapy for localized prostate cancer. *Rev Urol.* 2004;6(suppl 8):S24–S31.

23. Rossi CJ Jr, Slater JD, Reyes-Molyneux N, et al. Particle beam radiation therapy in prostate cancer: is there an advantage? *Semin Radiat Oncol.* 1998;8(2):115–123.

24. Slater JM, Archambeau JO, Miller DW, Notarus MI, Preston W, Slater JD. The proton treatment center at Loma Linda University Medical Center: rationale for and description of its development. *Int J Radiat Oncol Biol Phys.* 1992;22(2):383–389.

25. Slater JD, Yonemoto LT, Rossi CJ Jr, et al. Conformal proton therapy for prostate carcinoma. *Int J Radiat Oncol Biol Phys.* 1998;42(2):299–304.

26. Slater JD, Rossi CJ Jr, Yonemoto LT, et al. Proton therapy for prostate cancer: the initial Loma Linda University experience. *Int J Radiat Oncol Biol Phys.* 2004;59(2):348–352.

27. Zietman AL, DeSilvio ML, Slater JD, et al. Comparison of conventional-dose vs high-dose conformal radiation therapy in clinically localized adenocarcinoma of the prostate: a randomized controlled trial. *JAMA.* 2005;294(10):1233–1239.

28. Abramowitz MC, Li T, Buyyounouski MK, et al. The Phoenix definition of biochemical failure predicts for overall survival in patients with prostate cancer. *Cancer.* 2008;112(1):55–60.

29. Zietman AL, Bae K, Slater JD, et al. Randomized trial comparing conventional-dose with high-dose conformal radiation therapy in early-stage adenocarcinoma of the prostate: long-term results from proton radiation oncology group/american college of radiology 95–09. *J Clin Oncol.* 2010;28(7):1106–1111.

30. Talcott JA, Rossi C, Shipley WU, et al. Patient-reported long-term outcomes after conventional and high-dose combined proton and photon radiation for early prostate cancer. *JAMA.* 2010;303(11):1046–1053.

31. Mendenhall NP, Li Z, Morris CG, et al. Early GI and GU toxicity in three prospective trials of proton therapy for prostate cancer. *Int J Radiat Oncol Biol Phys.* 2009;75(3) (suppl):S11–S12.

32. Hara I, Murakami M, Kagawa K, et al. Experience with conformal proton therapy for early prostate cancer. *Am J Clin Oncol.* 2004;27(4):323–327.

33. Mayahara H, Murakami M, Kagawa K, et al. Acute morbidity of proton therapy for prostate cancer: the Hyogo Ion Beam Medical Center experience. *Int J Radiat Oncol Biol Phys.* 2007;69(2):434–443.

34. Fowler JF. The radiobiology of prostate cancer including new aspects of fractionated radiotherapy. *Acta Oncol.* 2005;44(3):265–276.

35. Constable IJ. Proton irradiation therapy for ocular melanoma. *Trans Ophthalmol Soc U K.* 1977;97(3):430.

36. Gragoudas ES, Goitein M, Verhey L, et al. Proton beam irradiation of uveal melanomas. Results of 5 ½-year study. *Arch Ophthalmol.* 1982;100(6):928–934.

37. Munzenrider JE, Austin-Seymour M, Blitzer PJ, et al. Proton therapy at Harvard. *Strahlentherapie.* 1985; 161(12):756–763.

38. Levy RP, Fabrikant JI, Frankel KA, Phillips MH, Lyman JT. Charged-particle radiosurgery of the brain. *Neurosurg Clin N Am.* 1990;1(4):955–990.

39. Steinberg GK, Fabrikant JI, Marks MP, et al. Stereotactic heavy-charged-particle Bragg-peak radiation for intracranial arteriovenous malformations. *N Engl J Med.* 1990;323(2):96–101.

40. Bush DA, Slater JD, Bonnet R, et al. Proton-beam radiotherapy for early-stage lung cancer. *Chest.* 1999;116(5):1313–1319.

41. Bush DA, Slater JD, Garberoglio C, Yuh G, Hocko JM, Slater JM. A technique of partial breast irradiation utilizing proton beam radiotherapy: comparison with conformal x-ray therapy. *Cancer J.* 2007;13(2):114–118.

42. Brenner DJ. Hypofractionation for prostate cancer radiotherapy–what are the issues? *Int J Radiat Oncol Biol Phys.* 2003;57(4):912–914.

43. Kupelian PA, Thakkar VV, Khuntia D, Reddy CA, Klein EA, Mahadevan A. Hypofractionated intensity-modulated radiotherapy (70 gy at 2.5 Gy per fraction) for localized prostate cancer: long-term outcomes. *Int J Radiat Oncol Biol Phys.* 2005;63(5):1463–1468.

44. Kupelian PA, Willoughby TR, Reddy CA, Klein EA, Mahadevan A. Hypofractionated intensity-modulated radiotherapy (70 Gy at 2.5 Gy per fraction) for localized prostate cancer: Cleveland Clinic experience. *Int J Radiat Oncol Biol Phys.* 2007;68(5):1424–1430.

45. Macías V, Biete A. Hypofractionated radiotherapy for localised prostate cancer. Review of clinical trials. *Clin Transl Oncol.* 2009;11(7):437–445.

46. Soete G, Arcangeli S, De Meerleer G, et al. Phase II study of a four-week hypofractionated external beam radiotherapy regimen for prostate cancer: report on acute toxicity. *Radiother Oncol.* 2006;80(1):78–81.

47. Fowler JF, Nahum AE, Orton CG. Point/Counterpoint. The best radiotherapy for the treatment of prostate cancer involves hypofractionation. *Med Phys.* 2006;33(9):3081–3084.

48. Kuban DA, Tucker SL, Dong L, et al. Long-term results of the M. D. Anderson randomized dose-escalation trial for prostate cancer. *Int J Radiat Oncol Biol Phys.* 2008;70(1):67–74.

49. Suit H, Kooy H, Trofimov A, et al. Should positive phase III clinical trial data be required before proton beam therapy is more widely adopted? No. *Radiother Oncol.* 2008;86(2):148–153.

50. Suit H. The Gray Lecture 2001: coming technical advances in radiation oncology. *Int J Radiat Oncol Biol Phys.* 2002;53(4):798–809.

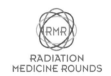

Proton Radiotherapy in Pediatric Malignancies

Sean M. McBride* and Torunn I. Yock

Massachusetts General Hospital, Boston, MA

■ ABSTRACT

Proton radiotherapy is a critical new treatment modality in the world of pediatric malignancies. The ability of proton radiotherapy to reduce significant dose to normal structures brings with it the promise of reduced long-term side effects. This is increasingly important in the pediatric population, where long-term survivors are quite common. A variety of data argues for the benefits of proton radiotherapy in the treatment of ependymoma, medulloblastoma, glioma, craniopharyngioma, germ cell tumors, retinoblastoma, rhabdomyosarcoma, and Ewing's sarcoma.

■ INTRODUCTION

Radiation is a critical component in the multi-modal treatment of many pediatric malignancies. Approximately 12,000 cases of childhood cancer are diagnosed every year. In children, the hematologic malignancies have the highest incidence followed by central nervous system (CNS) tumors, the most common solid malignancy in this population. The refinement in chemotherapeutic regimens, improvement in surgical techniques, and advances in radiation therapy technology have led to significant increases in the percentage of children surviving these diseases; overall survival at 5 years in all pediatric cancer patients has increased from 39% in 1960

*Corresponding author, Department of Radiation Oncology, Massachusetts General Hospital, Boston, MA 02114

E-mail address: smcbride@lroc.harvard.edu

Radiation Medicine Rounds 1:3 (2010) 491–510.
DOI: 10.5003/2151–4208.1.3.491

to more than 80% in 2004 (1). This dramatic improvement in outcomes has forced clinicians to reckon with the late treatment effects of these now curative therapies. Oeffinger et al. looked at 10,000 survivors of childhood cancer and found an exceedingly high prevalence of second cancers, cardiovascular disease, renal dysfunction, severe musculoskeletal problems, and endocrinopathies (2). The incidence of these chronic diseases in survivors does not appear to plateau with time.

Because of these late term effects, there is increasing interest in the use of proton therapy in the treatment of pediatric cancers. Already, with the widespread use of CT- and MRI-guided treatment, the accuracy of photon-based radiotherapy (RT) has increased (3). However, because of the physical properties associated with proton beam RT, they offer an additional benefit in reducing integral dose and thus acute and late toxicities.

Protons, and other charged particles, will deposit the vast majority of their dose at tumor depth. Only a small amount of energy is lost proximal to the tumor. Moreover, distal to the tumor volume, the dose deposited falls off completely, eliminating exit dose to the patient's normal tissues. In comparison, photons generally have a higher entrance dose and an exit dose. The proton's Bragg peak (Figure 1) is what give's proton particle radiation it's favorable dose distribution. Because the vast amount of dose is delivered across such a short distance, in order to adequately cover tumor volumes, multiple proton beams of various energies are used to create a homogenous dose distribution (Figure 1). Overall, this decreased dose both proximally and distally leads to greater sparing of normal tissue structures.

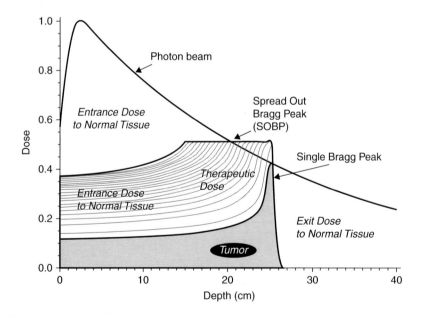

FIGURE 1

This is a graphical representation of the Bragg peak; the property of proton therapy that allows for steep dose drop off distal to the target. The use of multiple Bragg peaks allows for the treatment of a discrete target.

The acute toxicities that may be prevented by using proton RT are myriad and depend, in part, on the location of the tumor. For tumors of the head and neck, proton therapy may allow for a consequent reduction in alopecia, dermatitis, folliculitis, conjunctivitis, otitis externa, and pharyngitis. By using thoracic irradiation, the common acute side effects include esophagitis, pericarditis, dysphagia, and pneumonitis (which may be delayed up to 1 year). Finally, given that CNS disease is the most common solid malignancy in the pediatric population, protons may help to mitigate the nausea, vomiting, headache, and other neurologic sequelae that can accompany any type of cranial irradiation.

The long-term toxicities from RT, most especially neurocognitive changes and the risk of radiation-induced secondary malignancies, can be quite morbid. The impact of late side effects can be particularly burdensome in the pediatric population, both owing to the long lifespan after cure of the initial malignancy, and due to the fact that radiation to developing tissues will stunt further growth and development in a dose-dependent manner. Those are the long-term effects of cranial or craniospinal irradiation (CSI) that are often the most concerning to both families and physicians. Growth deficiencies, hearing deficits, and cognitive delay are often seen with traditional photon cranial RT. The spinal portion of the photon radiation can also cause morbidity in the organs receiving exit dose such as the heart, lungs, bowel, and uterus and ovaries (4,5).

There is a striking relationship between the volume (and dose) of photon cranial radiation and the magnitude of decline in later cognitive function (6); this relationship also holds for rates of secondary malignancy (7). Various estimates place the percentage of patients with secondary malignancy at near 20% with a time lag of between 10 and 50 years after initial treatment, although rates of second tumor induction also depend on a variety of host factors that include age at time of treatment, chemotherapy used, gender, and genetic predisposition. It is in reducing the incidence of these

sequelae that proton RT, because of its decreased integral dose, may provide the most benefit.

The under-utilization of proton therapy in pediatric patients is largely because of the scarcity of the resource. For many academic and private medical centers, construction costs are often prohibitive. There are currently seven operational proton facilities in the United States. They include the Massachusetts General Hospital (MGH, Boston, MA), MD Anderson Cancer Center (Houston, TX), the Hospital of the University of Pennsylvania (Philadelphia, PA), the University of Florida (Jacksonville, FL), Loma Linda Medical Center (Loma Linda, CA), the Procure Proton Therapy Center (Oklahoma City, OK), and the Midwest Proton Radiotherapy Institute (Bloomington, IN). Although pediatric patients comprise a significant plurality of patients treated at these centers, a large number of adults are also on treatment, further reducing availability. However, more centers will be opening as early as the end of 2010 in Hampton, VA, and Chicago, IL. Washington University (St Louis, MO) expects to be treating with protons by 2011. Other institutions and practices are planning additional centers.

■ PEDIATRIC BRAIN TUMORS

Intracranial neoplasms are the most common solid malignancy of childhood. Within this group, low-grade glioma (LGG) is the most common pediatric CNS tumor, comprising approximately 35% to 50% of all intracranial lesions; this is followed, in order of decreasing frequency, by medulloblastoma, brainstem glioma, high-grade glioma, and ependymoma (8). The incidence of CNS tumors peak from ages 3 to 7. For some lesions, such as standard risk medulloblastomas, 5-year overall survival can approach 85% (9). However, this impressive success is tempered by the realization that for tumors such as pediatric high-grade gliomas long-term survival statistics are still quite abysmal (10). With the increasing success of therapy, the need to address late effects of treatment has become an important priority within the pediatric oncology community. Fortunately, the literature on the late effects of intracranial photon radiation is growing and can provide benchmarks of how we can improve on these rates with more focused techniques using proton RT.

Irradiation of CNS tumors in children can cause endocrine deficiencies from the effects on the hypothalamus and/or pituitary gland. The probability of endocrine dysfunction is directly proportional to the dose of radiation received. Growth hormone and thyroid hormone are most likely to be affected. Significant decreases in cortisol or sex hormone levels are less common but can also occur (6,11). Craniospinal photon irradiation carries with it the additional risk of damage to the thyroid gland, uterus, and ovaries, causing end organ–related dysfunction (4,12).

Significant ototoxicity is also a concern for children receiving cranial irradiation. This is usually the result of unintended dose to the cochlea with negative effects being synergized by the use of ototoxic platinum chemotherapies. Furthermore, younger patients are at greater risk for radiation-induced ototoxicity than older patients (13). Many pediatric brain tumor patients receive cisplatin or carboplatin in the course of treating their tumor. Packer et al. reports that with concurrent cisplatin/vincristine and CSI, there is a 47.6% rate of grade 3 or 4 ototoxicity (14). Data extrapolated from nasopharyngeal cancer in adults suggests that the risk of ototoxicity increases substantially with doses above 50 Gy to the inner ear and cochlea (15). Hua and Merchant et al. have shown that radiation doses of less than 35 Gy to the cochlea generally do not have any clinically measurable effect provided platinum is not given. However, there is an increased frequency of negative effects when doses above 35 Gy are given (16).

The neurocognitive sequelae of cranial irradiation are often of greatest concern to patient, family, and physician. A pervasive year-by-year decline in intellectual functioning, often measured by the Wechsler Intelligence Scales for Children (WISC-R), has been consistently noted in the literature (17,18). Although intelligence quotient (IQ) tests measure global intellectual functioning, the cognitive deficits are particularly severe in tasks related to sustained attention, processing speed, and working memory (19,20). Radiation-related changes in myelination patterns are thought to contribute to the global decline in cognitive functioning (21). It is important to note that the volume of irradiated tissue is correlative with the degree of intellectual dysfunction (22). Although radiation clearly plays a significant role in cognitive delay, it has also been shown that the tumor itself, hydrocephalus, and surgery also contribute to decreased cognitive functioning relative to peers.

Regardless of the sources of neurocognitive decline, if significant, this late effect will often require a variety of educational and therapeutic interventions for appropriate management. Because the particle properties of protons reduce the volume of irradiated tissue, it is thought that proton-based treatments would carry with them a significantly reduced incidence of morbid late-term effects. Multiple dosimetric studies have been published in support of such a conclusion. One particularly striking example is from Merchant et al. (23). The authors used *in silico* dosimetric modeling to compare proton and photon plans on pediatric patients with intracranial lesions, including optic pathway glioma (ten), medulloblastoma (ten), craniopharyngioma (ten), and infratentorial ependymoma (ten). Dose cognitive effect models developed based on photon dosimetry, age, and neurocognitive changes in children were then used to estimate the likely detriment to IQ score over the long term (23). Large normal tissue volumes like the supratentorium and temporal lobes were exposed to significantly low and intermediate doses with proton therapy plans. Their models thus predicted that this relative sparing would lead to a statistically significant increase in IQ scores for the group of patients treated with protons versus photons.

Medulloblastoma

Medulloblastoma is the most common malignant CNS tumor of childhood. It accounts for approximately 20% to 30% of all brain tumors in the first decade of life with a median age of presentation of 6 to 7 years. The tumor is composed of immature, small round blue cells and arises within the posterior fossa (PF) (24). Approximately 30% to 40% of patients have cerebrospinal fluid (CSF) dissemination at the time of diagnosis. Poor prognostic factors include male sex, anaplastic or large cell histology, and CSF dissemination. Based, in part, on these prognostic factors and the extent of resection, patients are then categorized as standard risk or high risk (25). These risk categories dictate treatment course. Survival for standard risk patients approaches 80% to 85% (14), whereas survival for high risk disease can range from 50% to 70+% (25).

The mainstay therapy for either risk group remains surgical resection, followed by CSI and boost to the tumor bed as well as a platinum-based chemotherapy. One of the more common regimens, based on CCG 9892, is weekly vincristine during RT followed by vincristine, cisplatin, and CCNU for eight additional cycles (26). An additional option, outlined in the UKCCSG PNET 3 trial, is for preradiation chemotherapy to include four cycles alternating between vincristine, etoposide, carboplatin and then vincristine, etoposide, and cyclophosphamide. Compared to radiation alone, this resulted in a significant increase in 5-year event-free survival, 74.2% versus 59.8% (27). The latter option is common practice in Europe. In the infant population, a variety of chemotherapeutic regimens are tried after surgery in order to delay or obviate the need for adjuvant radiation (28). Children under 3 years are not given CSI RT because of its devastating late effects, but many regimens do incorporate focal field irradiation to help achieve local control.

CSI is given in both the standard and high-risk groups for children above 3 years of age—generally 23.4 Gy in the former and 36 Gy in the latter. Proton CSI is administered with children in either the prone or supine position depending on the center's immobilization and treatment techniques. For younger children, anesthesia may be necessary. Because precise immobilization is critical in intracranial tumors, a propofol-based anesthesia regimen is often used if positioning cannot be guaranteed; an aquaplast mask is standard in all patients. Data suggests that this type of anesthesia, repeatedly used for proton administration, is safe in children as young as 1 to 4 years of age (29). The spine is treated with two to three posterior fields that encompass the entirety of the vertebral bodies to avoid differential growth abnormalities and scoliosis. In older children who have completed bone growth, the thecal sac alone is targeted, which allows better sparing of the bone marrow in the vertebral bodies. The whole brain is treated with two posterior oblique fields in order to spare the lenses and sinuses, which in young children may not be pneumatized. CSI is then followed by a PF or involved field (IF) boost to doses of 54 to 55.8 GyE. The PF or IF is typically boosted to 54 Gy using two posterior oblique along with 1 PA field. In high risk patients, metastatic lesions are often brought to 45 to 54 GyE depending on location.

Proton Literature

There are data that argue in favor of the dosimetric superiority of protons over photons in the treatment of medulloblastoma. St. Clair et al. looked at isodose distributions and DVHs for a standard craniospinal axis irradiation and a PF boost using conventional 4 and 6 MV x-rays (30). This was compared with both an intensity-modulated radiation therapy (IMRT) for the same and whole brain irradiation using opposed lateral 160 MeV proton fields matched to a posterior-anterior proton spine field along with a PF boost using three field conformal protons. The test case was a 43-month-old boy who was sedated and scanned in the prone position. The most significant dose sparing of the cochlear apparatus and pituitary occurred with conformal protons. For instance, 90% of the cochlear volume was projected to receive 101.2% of the PF boost dose from conventional technique x-rays, 33.4% for IMRT, and 2.4% for protons. For the pituitary, the dose to 90% of the gland was 62.7% for x-rays, 19.3% for IMRT, and 0.1% for protons. Overall, conformal protons allowed for the greatest reduction in dose to all of the nontarget tissues outlined. These tissues, in addition to the aforementioned, included the hypothalamus, temporomandibular joints, parotid glands, and pharynx. Lee et al. also found an advantage to proton RT compared with photon or electron techniques (31).

Although the aforementioned data is *in silico* in nature, there is in vivo human data that the dose distributions described, namely the rapid fall-off distally, are accurate. This was convincingly outlined by Krejcarek et al. (32) and Gensheimer et al. (33). Radiation therapy to bone marrow can cause fatty replacement, which is well demonstrated on T1-weighted MR images. The authors

used this phenomenon to demonstrate (in vivo) the dosimetry of proton RT. The Krejcarek article evaluated the radiographic appearance of the vertebral bodies in children after CSI. The patients included 13 adolescents aged 12 to 18 years who had reached their maximal or near maximal height. Six of these patients had medulloblastoma. For older patients who have attained adult height, one is able to spare half of the vertebral body. The authors then looked to see if fatty marrow replacement occurred only in the posterior portion of the body that was irradiated. In the nine evaluable patients, all nine MRI images demonstrated a sharp demarcation of T1-weighted signal in the posterior portion of body suggesting significant sparing of the anterior portion owing to distal dose drop-off (Figure 2).

The aforementioned four studies demonstrate that proton RT, because of its reduction in the

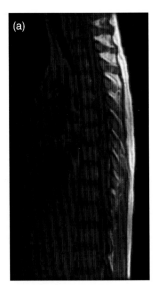 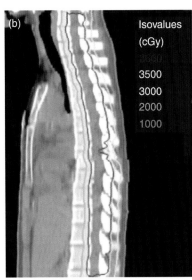 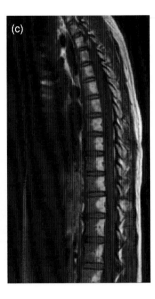

Isovalues
(cGy)

3500
3000
2000
1000

FIGURE 2
A 14-year-old girl with supratentorial primitive neuroectodermal tumor: craniospinal irradiation prescribed to the thecal sac and exiting nerve roots only. (a) T1-weighted magnetic resonance image 1 week before radiation treatment. (b) Computed tomography–proton radiotherapy treatment plan. (c) T1-weighted magnetic resonance image showing hyperintense fatty changes in posterior aspect of vertebral bodies 1 month after completion of proton radiotherapy.

dose of normal tissue irradiated, is highly likely to be capable of decreasing the frequency of late effects of therapy.

In addition to reducing the human cost of treatment-related side effects in medulloblastoma, there is evidence that proton RT is more cost effective than photon RT. Lundkvist et al. used a Markov simulation model to determine total lifetime costs for a cohort of 5-year-old medulloblastoma patients treated with protons and photon (34). They estimated that proton therapy would reduce total cost of caring for a child by €23,600.

Ependymoma

Approximately 200 children per year are diagnosed with ependymoma, encompassing approximately 8% to 10% of all pediatric CNS malignancies. Most children are diagnosed between ages 4 and 6; however, 25% to 40% are under 3 years. Ependymomas arise from the neuroepithelial lining of the ventricles and brain. The vast majority, approximately two-thirds, originate in the fourth ventricle. Biologically, one often sees overexpression of the EGF receptors *erbB-2* and *erbB-4*. The two primary histologic subgroups are anaplastic ependymoma and ependymoma, with the former portending a worse prognosis. Relapse, if it occurs, is primarily local. However, metastatic CNS relapse occurs in up to 25% of patients. These are more common in infratentorial and high-grade lesions.

The ability of surgeons to achieve a gross total resection (GTR) is the most critical prognostic factor. Recent data from St. Jude's Children's Research Hospital argues for the importance of both maximally safe surgical resection and radiation in achieving cure in this disease (35). They treated 153 patients with localized ependymoma from 1997 to 2007; 87 patients had anaplastic histology. The vast majority of tumors were infratentorial and most patients underwent GTR. They then received photon RT doses of 59.4 Gy or 54 Gy prescribed to a 1 cm margin around the

target volume. Overall survival at 5 years was 93% for patients achieving a GTR and 52.4% for those with a near-total or subtotal resection. Patients with anaplastic histology fared worse than their differentiated (grade II) counterparts, with a 5-year overall survival of 78.3% versus 91.9%. On multivariate analysis, the factors most predictive of overall survival included grade, extent of resection, and ethnic origin.

Radiation is also a critical component of treatment for ependymoma. Dose ranges from 54 Gy to 60 Gy to the postoperative tumor bed or residual disease with a 1-cm margin for clinical target volume (CTV). As is the case with many pediatric CNS malignancies, alternatives are sought to spare very young children from the deleterious effects of radiation. The current lower age limit for Children's Oncology Group (COG) ependymoma protocols is 1 year of age. There are data that suggest chemotherapy can be used to delay RT for more than 1 year (36).

Proton Literature

The MGH recently reported on the early outcomes for a series of 17 pediatric ependymoma patients treated with proton therapy between 2000 and 2006 (37). Dose was prescribed to the gross tumor volume (GTV) plus a 1-cm margin. Median prescribed dose was 55.8 cobalt gray equivalents (CGE; range, 52.2–59.4 CGE). Median age of the patients was 3.6 years. Thirteen patients had GTR; seven patients had anaplastic disease. Overall survival at a median follow-up of 26 months from the start of radiation was 89%; there were two local and one distant recurrences. IMRT plans were generated for two representative cases, one infratentorial and one supratentorial. Compared with the IMRT plan, the conformal, four-field proton plan spared significantly more whole brain and temporal lobes (Figure 3). Proton therapy plans decreased dose to all normal critical structures including the brainstem, pituitary gland, optic chiasm, left cochlea, right cochlea, and hypothalamus relative to the representative IMRT plans. For instance, 5% and 50% of the pituitary received 16 Gy and 12 Gy

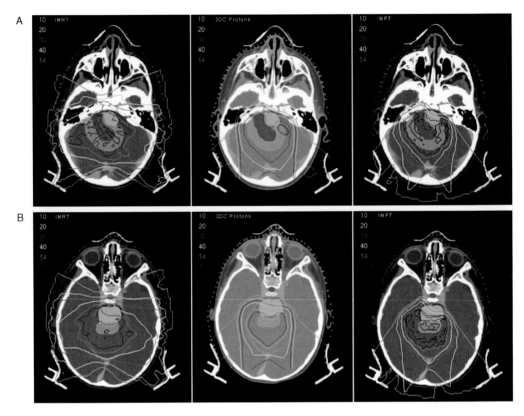

FIGURE 3
Intensity-modulated radiation therapy (IMRT), proton, and intensity-modulated proton therapy (IMPT) plans shown in the axial plane at the level of the (A) cochlea and (B) temporal lobes and pituitary gland. Gross Tumor Volume (GTV) is the smaller contoured volume contained within the Clinical Tumor Volume (CTV). Protons show improved sparing of the cochlea, cerebellum, pituitary gland, and temporal lobes. The IMPT plan shows superior proximal target conformity and further sparing of structures.

with the IMRT plans, respectively. With protons, this was reduced to less than 1 CGE. Overall, preliminary disease control is similar between protons and historic photon controls. The dosimetric parameters suggest a strong advantage for conformal proton therapy over photon IMRT.

Low-Grade Glioma

LGGs comprise approximately 40% of pediatric intracranial neoplasms. They can occur anywhere but will often require RT when they arise in the visual pathways, hypothalamus, thalami, or brainstem because of the morbidity of a surgical extirpation in these regions. Location appears to be an important prognostic factor in optic pathway gliomas, with chiasmal tumors faring worse than those confined to the optic nerve (38). Hemispheric LGGs generally carry an excellent prognosis with complete surgical resection (39). GTR is the most significant prognostic factor in hemispheric LGGs. In a series of 51 supratentorial juvenile pilocytic astrocytomas (JPA), those who had a GTR had a

10-year overall survival of 100% (40). Gliomas are the most common PF lesion. As is the case with hemispheric LGGs, the extent of surgical resection is important for prognosis, but cannot always be safely achieved in those tumors involving the brainstem.

Radiation treatment for unresectable or recurrent LGGs is often necessary. However, because of the indolent nature of these tumors and the age at which some of these patients present, lesions are often watched or treated with chemotherapy prior to definitive RT. In addition, we usually use radiation as a last resort with NF-1 patients because of the concern that RT may induce and second malignancy, and in many cases the tumors will become inactive when the child reaches adulthood. Furthermore, there is a fear that RT will lead to malignant progression in these NF-1 patients (41). Also, once NF-1 patients reach adulthood, their gliomas can enter a quiescent phase. However, RT should be used when chemotherapy fails and critical functions, such as vision, are at risk.

Chemotherapy is also used to delay RT in younger LGG patients; common regimens used include, vincristine/carboplatin, temazolomide, and vinblastine. St Jude's recently reported on its experience with radiation in 78 LGG patients treated between 1997 and 2006; 66 patients had grade I disease. Most tumors were diencephalic. Thirty-five patients had a subtotal resection with the remainder having either only a biopsy or no surgical procedure. Conformal photon radiation was used to a dose of 54 Gy prescribed to the GTV plus a 1-cm margin. With a median follow-up of 89 months, 13 patients experienced disease progression. The overall survival at 5 years and 10 years was 98.5% and 95.9%, respectively. Vasculopathy developed in 5% and was more common in younger patients. The patients are being followed for late effects.

Proton Literature

Dosimetric comparisons of proton and photon-based treatment of LGGs in the pediatric population demonstrate a benefit to sparing normal tissues with protons (23,42,43). Loma Linda University Medical Center reported on seven patients with optic pathway gliomas that underwent proton RT. They computed proton and three-dimensional RT photon plans based on the same CT data set in all seven patients. GTVs were delineated in all cases with dose of 54 CGE prescribed to the GTV plus a 0.5 to 1-cm margin. Proton plans contained four to nine coplanar and non–coplanar fields. Photon plans contained a median of six fields. Calculation of doses to normal tissue structures for both larger and smaller tumors showed that proton treatment outperformed photon three-dimensional RT in reducing dose to normal tissue. For instance, proton plans reduced doses to the contralateral optic nerve, chiasm, and pituitary gland by 47%, 11%, and 13%, respectively. Proton plans also reduced dose to the temporal lobes by 39%, which is believed to be very important for preserving neurocognitive functioning and memory. Importantly, target volume conformity was similar between three-dimensional photons and protons.

The same group from Loma Linda reported on outcomes in 27 pediatric LGG patients treated with proton RT from 1991 to 1997 at their facility (44). Twenty-five percent of tumors were located in the cerebral hemispheres, fifty-six percent in the diencephalon, and nineteen percent in the brainstem. Disease was biopsy-confirmed in 23 of 27 patients; grade II LGG was confirmed in 39% of patients and grade I in the remainder. Proton radiation was either administered adjuvantly (44%) or as salvage therapy at the time of recurrence (56%). Dose was administered to the CTV in 1.8 CGE fractions to a mean prescribed dose of 55.2 CGE. Mean follow-up was 3.3 years (0.6 to 6.8 years). Six of twenty-seven patients experienced local failure, all within the irradiated field, and four of twenty-seven died of their disease. Overall, 86% of patients with hemispheric lesions and 93% with central tumors were alive at the time of last follow-up. Local control for the hemispheric lesions was 71% versus 87% for central lesions. As predicted, patients with brainstem gliomas fared worse with local control rates of 60% at time of last follow-up. Acute side effects were minimal. One patient with neurofibromatosis developed Moyamoya syndrome. To date, no patients have experienced a significant decline in performance status.

Craniopharyngioma

Craniopharyngiomas are benign, partially cystic tumors of epithelial origins. They arise from remnants of the Rathke's pouch with most lesions being located in the suprasellar region. They represent 5% to 10% of intracranial lesions in children aged 5 to 14 years and commonly present with visual field disturbances and endocrine abnormalities (45). Treatment often involves resection, with GTR generally thought curative. Approximately 70% of craniopharyngiomas are amenable to complete surgical excision but radical excision can result in significant morbidities. There is a more recent trend to perform biopsy only or limited resection to debulk the tumor or cyst with planned definitive RT. Definitive radiation is recommended in the setting of gross residual disease after surgery (46).

St. Jude's reported on their experience with adjuvant radiation of craniopharyngioma in pediatric patients with a median age of 8.6 years (47). Median duration of follow-up was 72.7 months for surviving patients. Twenty-three patients received RT either adjuvantly or at relapse using a variety of techniques including radiosurgery (20–22 Gy × 1), fractionated EBT (54–55.8 Gy in 1.8 Gy fractions), and intracystic P-32 implantation. For the 15 patients treated with surgery initially, eight achieved GTR and seven STR. Nine patients recurred or progressed, with eight requiring salvage radiation. Fifteen patients underwent limited surgery (two with biopsy and the remainder with STR) and subsequently received definitive RT. Only one patient died of disease with the remainder still alive at time of last follow-up. The

authors concluded that STR followed by RT was comparable to GTR but that, surprisingly, the surgery group lost a mean of 9.8 IQ points compared with 1.25 points in the surgery-RT group. The surgery group also experienced increased neurologic, ophthalmic, and endocrine complications. These and other data have led many to conclude that radiation is effective in the immediate subtotal resection setting or as salvage in the treatment of craniopharyngiomas. Furthermore, this series supports the use of conservative surgery and RT over very morbid radical surgery for these tumors (48).

Proton Literature

There is a comparatively robust literature on proton therapy for craniopharyngioma. The Loma Linda group reported on 16 pediatric patients they treated with proton RT from 1991 to 2000, aged 3 to 17 years at diagnosis (49). Mean follow-up was 60.2 months. Four patients were treated with proton RT adjuvantly and 12 at the time of recurrence. Patients received doses ranging from 50.4 to 59.4 CGE. Beam arrangements consisted of right lateral, left lateral, and vertex fields. Twelve of 15 children were alive at last follow-up, with deaths occurring at 12, 52, and 120 months. All deaths occurred in patients who received repeat resection and salvage proton RT. Among the survivors, one developed panhypopituitarism at 36 months, one had a cerebrovascular accident at 34 months, and one developed a meningioma at 59 months after both photon external beam radiation therapy (EBRT) and salvage protons.

The MGH reported on a cohort of 15 pediatric and adult patients treated with combined photon-proton plans at the Harvard Cyclotron Laboratory between 1981 and 1988. The five children had a median age of 15.9 years. Median dose to the tumor was 56.9 CGE with a median proton component of 26.9 CGE; five patients received proton only therapy. Three-field techniques (laterals and a superior oblique) were used in all cases. Nine patients underwent proton/photon treatment after an STR, while six were treated at recurrence after multiple prior surgeries. Median observation period for surviving patients was 15.5 years. Actuarial 5- and 10-year overall survival rates were 93% and 72%, respectively. Four patients died of disease at 5, 5.6, 6.9, and 9.1 years after irradiation; all deaths were disease- or treatment-related. Before RT, all five of the pediatric patients required endocrine substitution. Four boys required testosterone substitution after RT. Of the five children, all graduated high school and three, at the time of publication, were attending college.

The MGH also reported on growth of the cystic components of craniopharyngiomas in 17 children before and after proton RT. The mean age at RT was 8.4 years. MRI or CT imaging was obtained before treatment, at week 1 and then week 3. Routine surveillance follow-up scans were also available. Ultimately, six patients needed intervention during treatment because of changes in cyst size. Four had cyst growth that went beyond the original CTV, necessitating re-planning. One patient actually had decrease in cyst size, allowing for decreased treatment volumes. Based on these observations, the authors concluded that routine surveillance imaging during treatment was warranted in these patients with a cystic component. Local control rates were 100% with a median follow-up on 40.5 months (range, 6–78 months) (50).

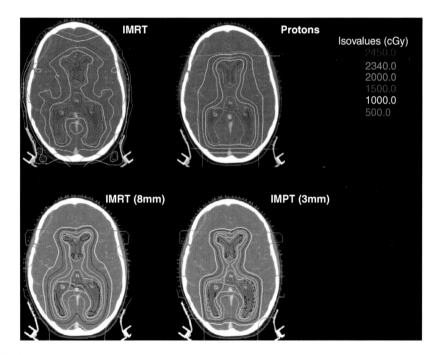

FIGURE 4

Axial CT images for whole-ventricular radition demonstrate superior dose delivery for proton radiation vs. intensity-modulated radiotherapy (IMRT). Intensity-modulated proton therapy (IMPT) with currently available IMPT (σ = 5–8 mm) shows some decrease in dose laterally to temporal lobes but results in increased "hot" and "cold" spots. More substantial normal tissue sparing with relatively homogenous target dose delivery can be achieved with a 3 mm σ. Protons = three-dimensional conformal proton therapy.

Intracranial Germ Cell Tumors

Compared to other pediatric intracranial neoplasms, germ cell tumors are more common in adolescents and collectively represent 3% to 5% of childhood CNS lesions. These tumors are typically located in the suprasellar region or within the pineal gland. Frequently localized, germ cell lesions are divided into two primary histologic categories: germinomas (more common) and nongerminomatous germ cell tumors (NGGCT). Germinomas are relatively responsive to EBRT; CSI was standard of care for many years, achieving cure in more than 90% of patients. However, because of its morbidity, CSI has been discarded in favor of whole ventricular system radiation (WVRT) followed by a boost to the IF in patients with localized disease. Pre-RT chemotherapy often involving etoposide and cisplatin in pure germinoma has also been used to good effect and may allow for a reduction in radiation dose (51). Treatment of NGGCT is far more controversial. A recently completed COG study (ACNS 0122) treated these patients with six cycles of induction carboplatin, ifosfamide, and etoposide followed by CSI to 36 Gy with an IF boost to 54 Gy. The European approach tends to focus on chemotherapy plus a more limited field approach to RT (52). The next COG study will evaluate a whole ventricle field with IF boost in nondisseminated cases in conjunction with chemotherapy and surgery.

Proton Literature

The MGH has recently reported on its series of 22 patients with germ cell tumors (13 with germinoma, 9 with NGGCT) treated from 1998 to 2007 with proton RT (52). Thirteen patients received CSI followed by IF boost, seven received WVRT followed by IF boost, one received treatment to IF only, and one received whole brain radiation therapy (WBRT) followed by IF boost. Dosimetric comparisons were made using a representative case that received WBRT followed by IF boost. IMRT, three-dimensional protons, and intensity-modulated proton therapy (IMPT) plans were compared (Figure 4). All NGGCT and 11 germinoma patients

received preradiation chemotherapy. At a median follow-up of 28 months (range, 13–97 months), local control, progression-free survival, and overall survival were 100%, 95%, and 100%, respectively. Two patients developed hypothyroidism after radiation; two developed growth hormone deficiency. In the dosimetric evaluations, similar tumor volume coverage was achieved with three-dimensional protons, IMRT, and IMPT. Proton therapy provided substantial normal tissue sparing compared with IMRT. For instance, the V30 for the right and left temporal lobes were 50.6% and 52.3% for IMRT. For proton RT, these numbers dropped to 8.9% and 9.7%, respectively. Overall, with similar local control and decreased integral dose to brain parenchyma, proton therapy offers a distinct advantage in the treatment of germ cell tumors.

■ NON-CNS PEDIATRIC TUMORS

The predominant sites of malignant pathology in the pediatric population are leukemia/lymphoma followed by CNS lesions. However, despite their decreased relative incidence, rhabdomyosarcoma (RMS; 3% of all pediatric malignancies), retinoblastoma (2%), and Ewing's sarcoma (2%) commonly require RT in the pediatric population. As with CNS lesions, the benefit of proton therapy resides in its ability to reduce acute and late-term sequelae by decreasing the volume of irradiated normal tissue. Proton RT could decrease integral dose to the bladder and rectum in the case of genitourinary (GU) RMS (53) as well as pelvic Ewing's sarcoma (31). Retinoblastoma and orbital RMS patients, because of the photon exit dose, may confront some of the same neurologic sequelae as patients treated for primary CNS lesions. Again, because of the Bragg peak, exit dose rapidly drops off and may spare children from these costly side effects.

Rhabdomyosarcoma

RMS is the most common soft tissue sarcoma of childhood. Of mesenchymal origin, two-thirds of RMS cases present before the age of 6 years; a second peak incidence occurs during adolescence (54). Head and neck is the most common site for RMS, with most tumors located in parameningeal regions (infratemporal fossa, middle ear canal, paranasal sinuses, nasal cavity, nasopharynx, mastoid area, and pterygopalatine fossa). The next three most common sites are GU (30%), extremity (15%), and trunk (15%). Embryonal and alveolar histologies are the two most common subtypes of RMS. The two major histologies have distinct genetic alterations associated with them and stark differences in prognosis.

Presentation obviously depends on location. GU tumors can present with painless hematuria, urinary frequency, or constipation. Orbital lesions can produce proptosis and ophthalmoplegia. Extremity and trunk lesions are often discovered when children or parents notice a painless, enlarging mass. RMS patients are risk stratified on the basis of stage and grouping. Staging is based on tumor size, positive lymph nodes, and favorable or unfavorable site. Favorable sites include nonparameningeal head and neck, GU (nonbladder, prostate), and biliary. Unfavorable sites include parameningeal, bladder/prostate, trunk, extremity, and retroperitoneum. Grouping is based on surgical outcome before starting any chemotherapy or radiation therapy (55). Patients are now categorized as low risk, intermediate risk, and high risk. The low-risk group is composed of both favorable and unfavorable sites with embryonal histologies that have been resected but also includes unresected orbital RMS. The intermediate-risk group includes nonmetastatic patients with unresected disease or patients with any alveolar histology. The high-risk group includes patients with metastatic disease (56).

Multimodal treatment is critical to achieving favorable outcomes in RMS patients. After surgical resection, vincristine, dactinomycin, and cyclophosphamide-based chemotherapeutic regimens form the backbone of treatment. Radiation doses depend on the risk group and extent of surgical resection. For low-risk patients, those with complete resection with negative surgical margins may often forgo RT; those with positive margins are treated to 36 Gy, while those with positive lymph nodes receive 41.4 Gy. Gross residual disease is treated to 50.4 Gy. In the intermediate-risk setting, doses that are similar save that complete resection still warrants 36 Gy regardless of margin status if delayed or up front and alveolar histology. Gross tumors in the orbit are treated to 45 Gy with concurrent chemotherapy after biopsy.

Proton Literature

The MGH reported on their experience treating seven children with orbital RMS using proton RT (57), with a dosimetric comparison between proton plans and photon IMRT. The seven patients were treated between 1995 and 2001 to a median dose of 46.6 CGE. Planning was CT-based with MRIs used to help further delineate target. Three patients had 20% of their dose delivered with photons. Median follow-up was 6.3 years (range, 3.5–9.7) with all patients alive at date of last visit. One patient who progressed through chemotherapy and who was under the age of 1 year suffered a local failure. He was salvaged with enucleation and stereotactic radiosurgery to the residual disease in the conus and remains NED. All others whose orbits were intact at the time of treatment had preserved vision. Two patients require lubricating drops on an ongoing basis. All patients had some degree of osseous hypoplasia. However, this late effect profile in this cohort compares very favorably to the late effects published in photon-treated cohorts in the literature (58). Importantly, no patient had endocrine abnormalities, which is a common side effect from photon radiation due to the exit dose to the hypothalamic pituitary axis. When making dosimetric comparisons between the proton and photon plans, there was dramatic sparing of the contralateral orbital structures with protons (Figure 5).

Since 1995, patients at the Paul Scherrer Institute in Villigen, Switzerland have been treated with spot scanning proton technology (59). They reported on their small series of 16 pediatric

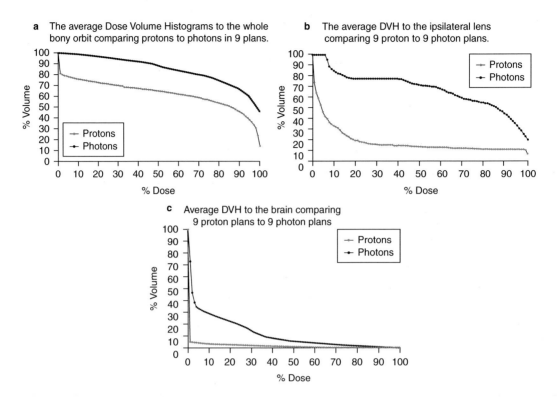

FIGURE 5

Comparison of average dose–volume histogram for all 7 patients (9 plans) between photons and protons for (a) bony orbital dose, (b) ipsilateral lens dose, and (c) incidental brain dose.

patients with sarcomas, 10 of whom had embryonal RMS. Tumor sites included parameningeal (seven), orbital (four), paraspinal (three), and prostate (one). Fourteen of these patients had biopsy only. The median dose of proton radiation was 50.0 CGE in 1.8 or 2 CGE fractions. At a median follow-up of 18.6 months (range, 4.3–70.8), 12 of the 16 patients had disease control (75%). Estimated progression-free survival at 1 and 2 years were 81.8% and 71.6%, respectively. Acute toxicities included severe lethargy in one female patient that resolved 6 weeks after proton RT. Two children experienced erythema and swelling of the lower eye-lid that persisted 8 weeks after proton RT.

More recently, MGH published its dosimetric comparison of proton versus photon therapy

in 10 patients with parameningeal RMS (59). The patients were all initially treated with protons. The authors then developed a matched photon IMRT plan for each patient. The primary parameningeal sites included the infratemporal fossa (six), paranasal sinuses (two), nasopharynx (one), and the middle ear (one). Intracranial extension was radiographically present in eight cases. The patients were treated with protons to a prescribed dose of 50.4 CGE to 52.2 CGE. When compared to IMRT, proton therapy provided significantly superior dose sparing for all examined organs. For example, the mean dose to the pituitary using protons compared to IMRT was 2,890 cGy and 4,320, respectively. The mean dose to the hypothalamus was 1,200 for proton therapy versus

2,480 for IMRT. The optic chiasm received a mean dose of only 1,770 cGy with protons compared to 3,690 with IMRT. Ipsilateral cochlea and mastoid were similarly spared. The MGH is set to report on the clinical outcome and late effects for 17 patients with parameningeal RMS treated at their institution between 1996 and 2005. The majority of these patients had embryonal histology and intracranial disease extension. The median prescribed was 50.4 CGE and, with a median follow-up of 4.4 years, the 3-year failure-free survival was 58% and overall survival, 61%. Of the 10 patients who had no evidence of recurrence at last follow-up, late effects included failure to maintain height velocity (n = 3), endocrinopathies (n = 2), mild facial hypoplasia (n = 7), visual or orbital complications (n = 3), failure of permanent tooth eruption (n = 3), multiple caries (n = 5), and chronic nasal/sinus congestion (n = 2). This side effect profile compares favorably with photon-based treatment (Childs S, Personal Communication, May, 2010).

Retinoblastoma

Retinoblastoma arises from the retinal neuroepithelium and, with approximately 200 cases per year in the United States, is the most common pediatric intraocular tumor. Two-thirds of children will present with unilateral, largely sporadic lesions, with the balance having a germline rotation in the *Rb* gene and will likely develop bilateral disease. The median age of diagnosis for sporadic lesions is 2 years. Hereditary lesions, caused by germline mutations in the *RB1* gene with subsequent loss of heterozygosity, are often bilateral and present earlier (often under 1 year) than their sporadic counterparts. Patients with a germline mutation in *RB1* are at greatly increased risk for secondary cancers in addition to retinoblastoma (60). Within radiation oncology, the Reese-Ellsworth classification system, designed to predict the risk of local recurrence, is often used in staging.

The clinical management of retinoblastoma has changed dramatically since the 1970s. For small tumors, a variety of options that are effective at locally controlling the lesion have been used. These include cryotherapy, thermotherapy, and photocoagulation. Cryotherapy is often used for tumors anterior to the equator of the eye. The latter two techniques are more commonly used for posterior pole tumors. Another option for small tumors is plaque RT.

For larger tumors or tumors that are adjacent to critical structures, enucleation is still considered to be the standard of care, especially when vision preservation is not feasible. For moderate or large sized tumors where globe preservation is possible and useful vision can be salvaged, neoadjuvant chemotherapy followed by local therapies is common practice.

The use of EBRT to achieve local control is well established. However, significant morbidities can result, including retinal injury, cataracts, dry eye, and even neuroendocrine dysfunction. Multiple series have demonstrated excellent local control achieved with photon EBRT. Hernandez et al. reported 78.5% local control in Reese-Ellsworth Group I-II patients treated to 45 Gy (61). Pradhan et al. demonstrated, at mean follow-up of 48.5 months, that 75% of patients remained without evidence of disease after EBRT (62). The majority (53%) still retained vision in the affected eye. Memorial Sloan Kettering reported an 83% local control rate at 8 years for patients with Group I-III Reese-Ellsworth retinoblastoma (63). St Jude's has demonstrated similar results at 10 years (64).

Proton Literature

Because of the known side effects of photon RT, the MGH, starting in 1986, began treating patients with retinoblastoma with proton RT (65). More recently, they published data regarding possible beam arrangement for proton RT. Most patients are treating in the supine position while under general anesthesia. A corneal suction cup was placed over the cornea of the affected eye in order to assure immobilization. Rotation of the cup would thus rotate the globe. Beam arrangements obviously depended on whether the tumor was temporal, central, or nasal in location. Plans were generated for the eye in three different positions: straight ahead, temporal rotation, and nasal rotation. All beam arrangements sufficiently covered the GTV and CTV. An anterolateral oblique approach with an intrarotated eye resulted in significant reduction of bony volume treated compared with a lateral beam arrangement. Overall, the authors concluded that proton therapy could reduce the risk of late-term effects, with a further decrease achievable with certain beam arrangements. Lee et al. compared dosimetry on plans for three retinoblastoma patients treated at MD Anderson. The authors compared three-dimensional conformal radiotherapy (3D-CRT) electron, 3D-CRT with a lateral beam, 3D-CRT with anterior and lateral beams with/without lens block, IMRT, and proton-based plans to a prescribed dose of 36 Gy in 18 fractions. Planning target volume (PTV) coverage using IMRT and three-dimensional RT with electrons was 95%. Other three-dimensional RT plans covered much less of the PTV. Protons were superior to all compared plans, covering 100% of the PTV. Lens sparing was superior with the three-dimensional RT electron, IMRT, and proton plans. The orbital bone received the lowest dose with the proton plan (31).

Ewing's Sarcoma

Ewing's sarcoma represents approximately 3% of all pediatric cancers and is the second most common bone malignancy after osteosarcoma with 70% of cases diagnosed before age 20. Ewing's sarcoma commonly arises in the long bones and pelvis but can occur anywhere and frequently presents with localized pain and swelling. Distant metastases, disease in the axial skeleton, large primary tumors, elevated lactate dehydrogenase, and older age are poor prognostic factors in Ewing's sarcoma. Treatment usually involves induction chemotherapy using an alternating combination of vincristine/adriamycin/cyclophosphamide and ifosfamide/etoposide. Local treatment is then typically initiated at week 12. Radiation and surgery are both viable local therapies, although some data

suggest superior local control with resection (66). Gross disease is treated to 55.8 Gy and microscopic disease is treated to 50.4 Gy. The 5-year event-free survival for localized disease ranges from 50% to 75% depending on the site with distal lesions doing better than pelvic or axial lesion. Metastatic disease fares worse, although lung-only metastatic disease is curable in up to 30% of the cases.

Proton Literature

The proton literature on Ewing's sarcoma is growing. Lee et al. included three patients with pelvic sarcoma in their dosimetric analysis and planned with three-dimensional RT, IMRT, and protons (31). All three techniques achieved adequate coverage. Notably, protons resulted in 0% ovarian irradiation. There were no significant differences in bowel and rectal dose; bladder dose was slightly lower with IMRT, whereas protons resulted in slightly lower dose to the pelvic bones. Gray et al. published a brief case report in 2009 on two pediatric patients treated with protons at the MGH for Ewing's sarcoma in the paranasal region (67). Case 1 was a 15-year-old female with Ewing's sarcoma of the left ethmoid sinus. She underwent consolidative proton radiation to 45 CGE in 1.8 CGE fractions to the prechemotherapy extent of disease with a cone down to residual disease to 59.4 CGE. She was free of disease at 2 years follow-up. The second case was one of a 17-year-old male with a left ethmoid Ewing's sarcoma with extension into the skull base. He had proton RT to 45 CGE with a cone down to 55.8 CGE to postchemotherapy volume.

Most recently, Rombi et al. reported in abstract form on 29 patients treated at the MGH (68). Ten of the patients received definitive proton RT with the remainder having it as postoperative treatment, two for salvage. The median prescribed dose was 52.8 CGE with a median follow-up of 26 months. The majority of cases had disease in the trunk and pelvis. Three-year overall survival, event-free survival, and local control were 84%, 63%, and 86%, respectively. Acute side effects included erythema and fatigue. However, three patients developed secondary acute myelogenous leukemia in the interim, which is a known side effect of the chemotherapy regimen used in Ewing's sarcoma, but this patient cohort will continue to be monitored closely.

■ CONTROVERSIES AND CONCLUSIONS

Besides the continued push and push-back regarding the need for large randomized controlled trials of proton RT (69), there is also significant controversy surrounding the issue of neutron scatter (70). Briefly, in order to provide adequate tumor coverage one of two techniques are used: (a) passively scattered large field proton RT, which is what the majority of proton centers are currently using, or (b) scanning beam technology. In the first option, the interaction of the protons with the scattering material can result in the production of high energy neutrons. The concern is that neutrons will significantly contribute to the risk of a radiogenic secondary malignancy. Initial estimates of the benefits of protons over photon radiation in secondary malignancy did not take into account the effects of secondary neutrons (71). Unfortunately, there exists no data on the actual carcinogenesis potential of high energy neutrons. Estimates are based on recommendations from the BEIR report (72) that err on the side of being conservative because these guidelines are used to limit exposures to radiation workers. Quality factors are loosely derived from relative biological effectiveness (RBE) estimates of cell kill and then increased for safety purposes.

In silico investigations into the incidence of secondary malignancies using passively scattered proton beams have been undertaken. The group at MD Anderson Cancer Center calculated doses to major organs and tissues from stray radiation following CSI with passively scattered proton therapy (73). They then used these dose predictions to estimate the risk of a fatal secondary radiogenic malignancy. From a CSI dose of 30.6 Gy with a boost of 23.4 Gy to the PF, they estimated stray radiation dose of 418 mSv, of which the vast majority was because of secondary neutron production outside of the body. They then estimated a 3.4% risk of a fatal secondary malignancy. Of importance, they note that this is an improvement on the Mirabell estimation of a fatal secondary cancer using photon IMRT.

Clinical data published in abstract form demonstrates that, in a cohort of adult and pediatric patients treated at the Harvard cyclotron matched with a SEER-database cohort, the use of passively scattered proton RT results in a lower rate of second tumor induction by at least half (74). This clinical data does not support the idea that neutron scatter increases the risk of second tumor induction in this population relative to photon controls.

In looking at pediatric malignancies as a whole, proton RT, because of its tight target delineation and ability to spare normal tissue, is ideal for the treatment of well-defined lesions in areas where late effects cause significant morbidity. As the number of proton centers in the United States continues to proliferate, it will be important to follow patients, and catalogue and report their side effect profiles and to find an appropriate comparison photon group in order to demonstrate the benefits of this therapy.

■ REFERENCES

1. Robison LL, Armstrong GT, Boice JD, et al. The Childhood Cancer Survivor Study: a National Cancer Institute-supported resource for outcome and intervention research. *J Clin Oncol.* 2009;27(14):2308–2318.
2. Oeffinger KC, Mertens AC, Sklar CA, et al. Chronic health conditions in adult survivors of childhood cancer. *N Engl J Med.* 2006;355(15):1572–1582.
3. Kooy HM, van Herk M, Barnes PD, et al. Image fusion for stereotactic radiotherapy and radiosurgery treatment planning. *Int J Radiat Oncol Biol Phys.* 1994;28(5):1229–1234.
4. Jakacki RI, Goldwein JW, Larsen RL, Barber G, Silber JH. Cardiac dysfunction following spinal irradiation during childhood. *J Clin Oncol.* 1993;11(6):1033–1038.
5. Jakacki RI, Schramm CM, Donahue BR, Haas F, Allen JC. Restrictive lung disease following treatment for malignant brain tumors: a potential late effect of craniospinal irradiation. *J Clin Oncol.* 1995;13(6):1478–1485.

6. Merchant TE, Conklin HM, Wu S, Lustig RH, Xiong X. Late effects of conformal radiation therapy for pediatric patients with low-grade glioma: prospective evaluation of cognitive, endocrine, and hearing deficits. *J Clin Oncol.* 2009;27(22):3691–3697.

7. Tubiana M. Can we reduce the incidence of second primary malignancies occurring after radiotherapy? A critical review. *Radiother Oncol.* 2009;91(1):4–15; discussion 1.

8. Ross JA, Olshan AF. Pediatric cancer in the United States: the Children's Oncology Group Epidemiology Research Program. *Cancer Epidemiol Biomarkers Prev.* 2004;13(10):1552–1554.

9. Gajjar A, Chintagumpala M, Ashley D, et al. Risk-adapted craniospinal radiotherapy followed by high-dose chemotherapy and stem-cell rescue in children with newly diagnosed medulloblastoma (St Jude Medulloblastoma-96): long-term results from a prospective, multicentre trial. *Lancet Oncol.* 2006;7(10):813–820.

10. Broniscer A, Gajjar A. Supratentorial high-grade astrocytoma and diffuse brainstem glioma: two challenges for the pediatric oncologist. *Oncologist.* 2004;9(2):197–206.

11. Heikens J, Ubbink MC, van der Pal HP, et al. Long term survivors of childhood brain cancer have an increased risk for cardiovascular disease. *Cancer.* 2000; 88(9):2116–2121.

12. Harden SV, Twyman N, Lomas DJ, Williams D, Burnet NG, Williams MV. A method for reducing ovarian doses in whole neuro-axis irradiation for medulloblastoma. *Radiother Oncol.* 2003;69(2):183–188.

13. Grewal S, Merchant T, Reymond R, McInerney M, Hodge C, Shearer P. Auditory late effects of childhood cancer therapy: a report from the Children's Oncology Group. *Pediatrics.* 2010;125(4):e938–e950.

14. Packer RJ, Sutton LN, Elterman R, et al. Outcome for children with medulloblastoma treated with radiation and cisplatin, CCNU, and vincristine chemotherapy. *J Neurosurg.* 1994;81(5):690–698.

15. Low WK, Toh ST, Wee J, Fook-Chong SM, Wang DY. Sensorineural hearing loss after radiotherapy and chemoradiotherapy: a single, blinded, randomized study. *J Clin Oncol.* 2006;24(12):1904–1909.

16. Hua C, Bass JK, Khan R, Kun LE, Merchant TE. Hearing loss after radiotherapy for pediatric brain tumors: effect of cochlear dose. *Int J Radiat Oncol Biol Phys.* 2008;72(3):892–899.

17. Spiegler BJ, Bouffet E, Greenberg ML, Rutka JT, Mabbott DJ. Change in neurocognitive functioning after treatment with cranial radiation in childhood. *J Clin Oncol.* 2004;22(4):706–713.

18. Ris MD, Packer R, Goldwein J, Jones-Wallace D, Boyett JM. Intellectual outcome after reduced-dose radiation therapy plus adjuvant chemotherapy for medulloblastoma: a Children's Cancer Group study. *J Clin Oncol.* 2001;19(15):3470–3476.

19. Huang E, Teh BS, Strother DR, et al. Intensity-modulated radiation therapy for pediatric medulloblastoma: early report on the reduction of ototoxicity. *Int J Radiat Oncol Biol Phys.* 2002;52(3):599–605.

20. Schatz J, Kramer JH, Ablin A, Matthay KK. Processing speed, working memory, and IQ: a developmental model of cognitive deficits following cranial radiation therapy. *Neuropsychology.* 2000;14(2):189–200.

21. Khong PL, Leung LH, Fung AS, et al. White matter anisotropy in post-treatment childhood cancer survivors: preliminary evidence of association with neurocognitive function. *J Clin Oncol.* 2006;24(6):884–890.

22. Merchant TE, Kiehna EN, Li C, et al. Modeling radiation dosimetry to predict cognitive outcomes in pediatric patients with CNS embryonal tumors including medulloblastoma. *Int J Radiat Oncol Biol Phys.* 2006; 65(1):210–221.

23. Merchant TE, Hua CH, Shukla H, Ying X, Nill S, Oelfke U. Proton versus photon radiotherapy for common pediatric brain tumors: comparison of models of dose characteristics and their relationship to cognitive function. *Pediatr Blood Cancer.* 2008;51(1):110–117.

24. Fossati P, Ricardi U, Orecchia R. Pediatric medulloblastoma: toxicity of current treatment and potential role of protontherapy. *Cancer Treat Rev.* 2009; 35(1):79–96.

25. McLean TW. Medulloblastomas and central nervous system primitive neuroectodermal tumors. *Curr Treat Options Oncol.* 2003;4(6):499–508.

26. Packer RJ, Goldwein J, Nicholson HS, et al. Treatment of children with medulloblastomas with reduced-dose craniospinal radiation therapy and adjuvant chemotherapy: a Children's Cancer Group Study. *J Clin Oncol.* 1999;17(7):2127–2136.

27. Taylor RE, Bailey CC, Robinson K, et al. Results of a randomized study of preradiation chemotherapy versus radiotherapy alone for nonmetastatic medulloblastoma: The International Society of Paediatric Oncology/United Kingdom Children's Cancer Study Group PNET-3 Study. *J Clin Oncol.* 2003;21(8): 1581–1591.

28. Heideman RL. Overview of the treatment of infant central nervous system tumors: medulloblastoma as a model. *J Pediatr Hematol Oncol.* 2001;23(5):268–271.

29. Buehrer S, Immoos S, Frei M, Timmermann B, Weiss M. Evaluation of propofol for repeated prolonged deep sedation in children undergoing proton radiation therapy. *Br J Anaesth*. 2007;99(4):556–560.

30. St Clair WH, Adams JA, Bues M, et al. Advantage of protons compared to conventional X-ray or IMRT in the treatment of a pediatric patient with medulloblastoma. *Int J Radiat Oncol Biol Phys*. 2004;58(3):727–734.

31. Lee CT, Bilton SD, Famiglietti RM, et al. Treatment planning with protons for pediatric retinoblastoma, medulloblastoma, and pelvic sarcoma: how do protons compare with other conformal techniques? *Int J Radiat Oncol Biol Phys*. 2005;63(2):362–372.

32. Krejcarek SC, Grant PE, Henson JW, Tarbell NJ, Yock TI. Physiologic and radiographic evidence of the distal edge of the proton beam in craniospinal irradiation. *Int J Radiat Oncol Biol Phys*. 2007;68(3):646–649.

33. Gensheimer MF, Yock TI, Liebsch NJ, et al. *In vivo* proton beam range verification using spine MRI changes. *Int J Radiat Oncol Biol Phys*. 2010;78(1):268–275.

34. Lundkvist J, Ekman M, Ericsson SR, Jönsson B, Glimelius B. Cost-effectiveness of proton radiation in the treatment of childhood medulloblastoma. *Cancer*. 2005;103(4):793–801.

35. Merchant TE, Li C, Xiong X, Kun LE, Boop FA, Sanford RA. Conformal radiotherapy after surgery for paediatric ependymoma: a prospective study. *Lancet Oncol*. 2009;10(3):258–266.

36. Duffner PK, Horowitz ME, Krischer JP, et al. The treatment of malignant brain tumors in infants and very young children: an update of the Pediatric Oncology Group experience. *Neuro-oncology*. 1999;1(2):152–161.

37. MacDonald SM, Safai S, Trofimov A, et al. Proton radiotherapy for childhood ependymoma: initial clinical outcomes and dose comparisons. *Int J Radiat Oncol Biol Phys*. 2008;71(4):979–986.

38. Wong JY, Uhl V, Wara WM, Sheline GE. Optic gliomas. A reanalysis of the University of California, San Francisco experience. *Cancer*. 1987;60(8):1847–1855.

39. Pollack IF, Claassen D, al-Shboul Q, Janosky JE, Deutsch M. Low-grade gliomas of the cerebral hemispheres in children: an analysis of 71 cases. *J Neurosurg*. 1995;82(4):536–547.

40. Forsyth PA, Shaw EG, Scheithauer BW, O'Fallon JR, Layton DD Jr, Katzmann JA. Supratentorial pilocytic astrocytomas. A clinicopathologic, prognostic, and flow cytometric study of 51 patients. *Cancer*. 1993;72(4):1335–1342.

41. Ishii N, Tada M, Hamou MF, et al. Cells with TP53 mutations in low grade astrocytic tumors evolve clonally to malignancy and are an unfavorable prognostic factor. *Oncogene*. 1999;18(43):5870–5878.

42. Fuss M, Hug EB, Schaefer RA, et al. Proton radiation therapy (PRT) for pediatric optic pathway gliomas: comparison with 3D planned conventional photons and a standard photon technique. *Int J Radiat Oncol Biol Phys*. 1999;45(5):1117–1126.

43. Yock TOJ, Yeap B, Tarbell NJ. Preliminary Report of Proton Radiotherapy in Low Grade Glioma. *Int J Radiat Oncol Biol Phys*. 2005;63:S443–S442.

44. Hug EB, Muenter MW, Archambeau JO, et al. Conformal proton radiation therapy for pediatric low-grade astrocytomas. *Strahlenther Onkol*. 2002;178(1):10–17.

45. Ohmori K, Collins J, Fukushima T. Craniopharyngiomas in children. *Pediatr Neurosurg*. 2007;43(4):265–278.

46. Kiehna EN, Merchant TE. Radiation therapy for pediatric craniopharyngioma. *Neurosurg Focus*. 2010;28(4):E10.

47. Merchant TE, Kiehna EN, Sanford RA, et al. Craniopharyngioma: the St. Jude Children's Research Hospital experience 1984–2001. *Int J Radiat Oncol Biol Phys*. 2002;53(3):533–542.

48. Stripp DC, Maity A, Janss AJ, et al. Surgery with or without radiation therapy in the management of craniopharyngiomas in children and young adults. *Int J Radiat Oncol Biol Phys*. 2004;58(3):714–720.

49. Luu QT, Loredo LN, Archambeau JO, Yonemoto LT, Slater JM, Slater JD. Fractionated proton radiation treatment for pediatric craniopharyngioma: preliminary report. *Cancer J*. 2006;12(2):155–159.

50. Winkfield KM, Linsenmeier C, Yock TI, et al. Surveillance of craniopharyngioma cyst growth in children treated with proton radiotherapy. *Int J Radiat Oncol Biol Phys*. 2009;73(3):716–721.

51. Aoyama H, Shirato H, Ikeda J, Fujieda K, Miyasaka K, Sawamura Y. Induction chemotherapy followed by low-dose involved-field radiotherapy for intracranial germ cell tumors. *J Clin Oncol*. 2002;20(3):857–865.

52. Macdonald SM, Trofimov A, Safai S, et al. Proton radiotherapy for pediatric central nervous system germ cell tumors: early clinical outcomes. *Int J Radiat Oncol Biol Phys*. 2010;[Epub ahead of print].

53. Cotter SE, Herrup DA, Adams J, et al. Clinical outcomes of proton radiotherapy for pediatric bladder/prostate rhabdomyosarcoma and a dosimetric comparison with intensity modulated radiotherapy. *Int J Radiat Oncol Biol Phys*. 2009;75:S511.

54. Punyko JA, Mertens AC, Baker KS, Ness KK, Robison LL, Gurney JG. Long-term survival probabilities for childhood rhabdomyosarcoma. A population-based evaluation. *Cancer.* 2005;103(7):1475–1483.

55. Rodeberg DA, Paidas CN, Lobe TL, et al. Surgical principles for children/adolescents with newly diagnosed rhabdomyosarcoma: a report from the Soft Tissue Sarcoma Committee of the Children's Oncology Group. *Sarcoma.* 2002;6(4):111–122.

56. Raney RB, Maurer HM, Anderson JR, et al. The Intergroup Rhabdomyosarcoma Study Group (IRSG): major lessons from the IRS-I through IRS-IV studies as background for the current IRS-V treatment protocols. *Sarcoma.* 2001;5(1):9–15.

57. Yock T, Schneider R, Friedmann A, Adams J, Fullerton B, Tarbell N. Proton radiotherapy for orbital rhabdomyosarcoma: clinical outcome and a dosimetric comparison with photons. *Int J Radiat Oncol Biol Phys.* 2005;63(4):1161–1168.

58. Oberlin O, Rey A, Anderson J, et al. Treatment of orbital rhabdomyosarcoma: survival and late effects of treatment–results of an international workshop. *J Clin Oncol.* 2001;19(1):197–204.

59. Kozak KR, Adams J, Krejcarek SJ, Tarbell NJ, Yock TI. A dosimetric comparison of proton and intensity-modulated photon radiotherapy for pediatric parameningeal rhabdomyosarcomas. *Int J Radiat Oncol Biol Phys.* 2009;74(1):179–186.

60. Kleinerman RA, Tarone RE, Abramson DH, Seddon JM, Li FP, Tucker MA. Hereditary retinoblastoma and risk of lung cancer. *J Natl Cancer Inst.* 2000; 92(24):2037–2039.

61. Hernandez JC, Brady LW, Shields JA, et al. External beam radiation for retinoblastoma: results, patterns of failure, and a proposal for treatment guidelines. *Int J Radiat Oncol Biol Phys.* 1996;35(1):125–132.

62. Pradhan DG, Sandridge AL, Mullaney P, et al. Radiation therapy for retinoblastoma: a retrospective review of 120 patients. *Int J Radiat Oncol Biol Phys.* 1997;39(1):3–13.

63. Blach LE, McCormick B, Abramson DH. External beam radiation therapy and retinoblastoma: long-term results in the comparison of two techniques. *Int J Radiat Oncol Biol Phys.* 1996;35(1):45–51.

64. Merchant TE, Gould CJ, Hilton NE, et al. Ocular preservation after 36 Gy external beam radiation therapy for retinoblastoma. *J Pediatr Hematol Oncol.* 2002;24(4):246–249.

65. Krengli M, Hug EB, Adams JA, Smith AR, Tarbell NJ, Munzenrider JE. Proton radiation therapy for retinoblastoma: comparison of various intraocular tumor locations and beam arrangements. *Int J Radiat Oncol Biol Phys.* 2005;61(2):583–593.

66. Krasin MJ, Rodriguez-Galindo C, Davidoff AM, et al. Efficacy of combined surgery and irradiation for localized Ewings sarcoma family of tumors. *Pediatr Blood Cancer.* 2004;43(3):229–236.

67. Gray ST, Chen YL, Lin DT. Efficacy of Proton Beam Therapy in the Treatment of Ewing's Sarcoma of the Paranasal Sinuses and Anterior Skull Base. *Skull Base.* 2009;19(6):409–416.

68. Rombi BDT, MacDonald SM, Yeap B, et al. Proton radiotherapy for pediatric Ewing's sarcoma: initial clinical outcome of 29 patients. In: Particle Therapy Co-operative Group, 48th Annual Meeting; September 29–October 3, 2009; Edition Heidelberg, Germany.

69. Goitein M, Cox JD. Should randomized clinical trials be required for proton radiotherapy? *J Clin Oncol.* 2008;26(2):175–176.

70. Hall EJ. The impact of protons on the incidence of second malignancies in radiotherapy. *Technol Cancer Res Treat.* 2007;6(4 suppl):31–34.

71. Miralbell R, Lomax A, Cella L, Schneider U. Potential reduction of the incidence of radiation-induced second cancers by using proton beams in the treatment of pediatric tumors. *Int J Radiat Oncol Biol Phys.* 2002; 54(3):824–829.

72. Monson RP. *Health Risks from Exposure to Low Levels of Ionizing Radiation: BEIR VII Phase 2.* Washington, DC: National Academies Press; 2006.

73. Taddei PJ, Mirkovic D, Fontenot JD, et al. Stray radiation dose and second cancer risk for a pediatric patient receiving craniospinal irradiation with proton beams. *Phys Med Biol.* 2009;54(8):2259–2275.

74. Chung CS KN, Yock Y, Tarbell NJ. Comparative analysis of second malignancy risk in patients treated with proton therapy versus conventional photon therapy. *Int J Radiat Oncol Biol Phys.* 2008;72:S8.

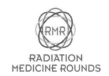

RADIATION
MEDICINE ROUNDS

Proton Therapy for Adult Brain Tumors and Base of Skull Tumors

Michelle Alonso-Basanta*

University of Pennsylvania Health System, Philadelphia, PA

■ ABSTRACT

Proton radiotherapy has been used in clinical practice for more than 50 years. As more centers are opened across the country and the world, it is becoming increasingly important to determine the effectiveness and feasibility of using protons. In no other site has proton therapy been more important than in the CNS. The following is a brief review of the current treatment rationale using protons for various tumors of the brain and base of skull.

Keywords: Proton, brain, base of skull, toxicity, AVMs, glioma, meningioma, pituitary adenoma, acoustic neuroma

In 2010, brain and other CNS tumors account for an estimated 22,020 new cases and an estimated 13,140 deaths (1). This group is very heterogeneous from benign tumors (e.g., pituitary adenomas and acoustic neuromas) to malignant tumors, most notably glioblastoma multiforme (GBM). Given this diversity in histology, it is important that each patient's case is reviewed and a treatment option is determined by a multidisciplinary team of experts including neurosurgeons, radiation oncologists, neuroradiologists and neuro-oncologists. Although various attempts have been made to minimize the role of radiation, the standard of care remains as surgical resection followed by radiation therapy ± chemotherapy depending on the histology (2,3).

Therefore, research has focused on the modality of radiation as well as the total dose and fractionation. In particular, given the increasing number of treatment centers in the United States (with more centers to open in the future), research has focused on proton therapy in the treatment of brain tumors and base of skull tumors.

The first proton references in the literature with regard to treating primary brain tumors date back to the 1960s in murine models (4–6) with

*Corresponding author, Department of Radiation Oncology, University of Pennsylvania Health System, Philadelphia, PA 19104
  E-mail address: michelleab@uphs.upenn.edu

Radiation Medicine Rounds 1:3 (2010) 511–522.
DOI: 10.5003/2151–4208.1.3.511

demosmedpub.com/rmr

early work in skull base tumors (7,8) and then moving toward intracranial tumors in the early 1970s (9). Colleagues in Uppsala Sweden in 1975 reported on the use of proton beam therapy in the postoperative setting in malignant glioma (10). The following is a brief overview of the advances to treatment in the brain and base of skull with a focus on the future for proton therapy.

■ BRAIN

Arteriovenous Malformations

In the benign setting, arteriovenous malformations (AVMs) have been treated with proton therapy since its early days in clinical use. Kiellberg reported in 1986 the use of stereotactic proton beam radiosurgery for AVMs in 709 patients (11). With a follow-up of 2 years, he reported a slightly lower threshold for proton injury than normal tissue. Further review of Dr. Kiellberg's cases at the Harvard Cyclotron was later reported in 2003 examining 1,250 patients treated between 1965 and 1993 (12). Median follow-up was 6.5 years. The median dose was 10.5 Gy with a treatment volume of 33.7 cm³. Permanent radiation-related deficits were seen in 4.1% of cases. They performed fitted logistic modeling, which showed that the complication risk was related to treatment dose and volume, thalamic or brainstem location, and patient age.

Given these risks, fractionated, stereotactic proton beam therapy has been reviewed (13,14). Colleagues in South Africa treated AVMs using hypofractionated proton radiotherapy in 64 patients and then grouped them according to volume (<14 cc and ≥14 cc). The mean dose delivered using a fixed horizontal 200 MeV proton beam was 17.37 cGyE (range 10.38–22.05) (14). Obliteration was seen in 67% for volumes below 14 cc and in 43% for volumes more than or equal to 14 cc. Three percent of patients developed acute grade IV complications with 23% experiencing transient effects and three patients experiencing permanent effects. For larger volume AVMs, this is a viable option.

Brain Tumors

Malignant brain tumors including grade I and II astrocytomas have traditionally been either observed or treated with radiation therapy alone depending on whether you are a "believer" or "nonbeliever." Radiation therapy has typically been given using a 3D conformal technique or through intensity-modulated radiation therapy (IMRT) using a number of fields and therefore increasing the integral dose to the body and other structures. However, for concave and convex tumors, these techniques have enabled better sparing of normal structures (15,16). Proton therapy has now taken center stage in regard to better spare normal brain and therefore improve upon neurocognitive deficits that have become an increasing focus not only on primary brain tumors but also on metastatic disease (17). Of importance is its role in the pediatric population where treatment of the CNS will have an impact on long-term sequelae (18). Figure 1 is an example of a patient treated with proton therapy for a low-grade astrocytoma.

At a mean follow-up of 3.3 years, a review of the first 27 patients treated at Loma Linda University Medical Center (LLUMC) to a target dose between 50.4 and 63 cGyE showed a local control rate of 87% and overall survival of 93% (19). Overall proton therapy was well tolerated. Twenty-eight patients at Loma Linda were identified as at risk for brain injury from treatment with protons (20). With a median follow-up of 25 months, four instances of treatment-related morbidity were identified and 41 instances of site-specific, disease-related morbidity were identified. Four patients had radiographic evidence of local failure. They concluded that early treatment-related morbidity associated with proton therapy was low however ongoing neurocognitive studies would ultimately dictate this. Current studies including a study at the University of Pennsylvania are examining the neurocognitive function of patients after proton therapy and comparing these to a retrospective cohort of patients treated with photons (www.clinicaltrials.gov).

A   Photons-IMRT   B   Protons

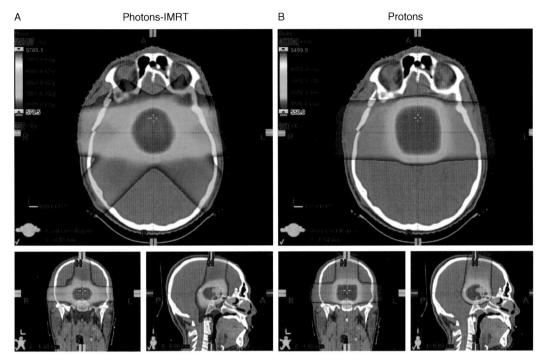

FIGURE 1
Patient with a low-grade glioma in the frontal lobe. (A) Intensity-modulated radiation therapy. (B) Proton radiation therapy.

In addition, as techniques in protons improve, we would expect that late sequelae will decrease. Colleagues at the Paul Scherrer Institute in Switzerland reviewed the use of a single dorsal field in treating the craniospinal axis in a single case study (21). They achieved a homogeneous dose and were able to minimize ventral dose while avoiding patching fields.

Dose escalation has been reported in this patient population with a dose of 68.2 cGyE using standard daily fractionation of 1.8 cGyE for grade 2 tumors (22). With a median follow-up of 61 months, the actuarial 5-year survival rate was 71% with median survival not reached. Tumor recurrence was not prevented or delayed compared to a similar series treated with photon irradiation.

There was evidence of radiation necrosis in the tumor specimen. There was no improvement in outcome.

The benefit of proton therapy in high-grade gliomas is somewhat controversial. There is evidence that malignant cells are at least 2 cm from the enhancing tumor on magnetic resonance imaging (MRI) (23,24) and, therefore, there is the question of "sparing" with protons. However, their use may be more valuable for dose escalation without decreasing the "margin" on treatment volumes as is now done on other studies (25). Colleagues in Japan are using protons as a concomitant boost for supratentorial GBM (26). All patients were treated to a total dose of 50.4 Gy with a concomitant boost with proton beams

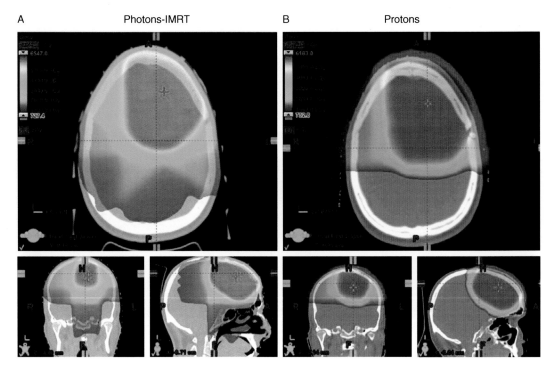

FIGURE 2
Patient with a recurrent glioblastoma multiforme. (A) Intensity-modulated radiation therapy. (B) Proton radiation therapy.

delivered to the enhanced area plus a 1-cm margin in the first half of the protocol (23.1 cGyE in 14 fractions) and to the enhanced volume alone in the latter half (23.1 cGyE in 14 fractions). The total dose delivered was 96.6 cGyE. The overall survival at 2 years was 45.3% with a median survival of 21.6 months. The 2-year progression-free survival rate was 15.5%. Figure 2 is an example of a high-grade glioma undergoing radiation therapy with protons and temozolomide.

Metastases

There is no current role for protons in brain metastases. Stereotactic radiosurgery (SRS) remains to be an acceptable and viable treatment for small lesions within the parenchyma of the brain. However, as these tumors become larger and the risk/benefit ratio shifts, the role of protons will become more important. Fractionated radiosurgery has already been implemented with multiple modalities for larger brain metastases (27).

■ BASE OF SKULL

Chordomas and Chondrosarcomas

The benefit of proton therapy has been best seen in chordomas and chondrosarcomas of the base of skull. Reports in 1982 showed that treatment of 10 patients to doses of 76 cobalt gray equivalent (CGE) was feasible without significant morbidity (28). Massachusetts General Hospital (MGH) reported on the use of fractionated proton radiation therapy in 1989 on 68 patients who received postoperative radiation therapy to a median dose of 69 CGE with a 5-year actuarial local control rate of 82% and disease-free survival of 76% (29). Temporal lobe damage was reported by the same institution in 1998 in 96 patients with chordomas and chondrosarcomas of the base of skull (30). All patients were treated to either 66.6 or 72 CGE with conventional fractionation. Ten patients developed temporal lobe damage with a cumulative damage incidence of 13.2% at 5 years. Despite the different temporal lobe damage rates related to age, tumor volume, number of surgical procedures prior to radiation therapy, and prescribed doses to the tumor, only gender was a significant predictor of damage ($P = 0.0155$) using a univariate (log rank) test. In a stepwise Cox regression that included gender as a variable, no other baseline variable improved the prediction of damage.

A review of cases at MGH published in 1999 showed a 10-year local control rate of combined proton-photon therapy that was highest for chondrosarcomas, intermediate for male chordomas, and lowest for female chordomas (94%, 65%, and 42%, respectively) (31). A similar review at LLUMC in 58 patients with skull base chordomas and chondrosarcomas treated to total doses between 64.8 and 79.2 CGE showed local control rates of 92% for chondrosarcoma and 76% for chordomas (32). Actuarial 5-year survival rates were 100% for patients with chondrosarcoma and 79% for patients with chordoma. Grade 3 and 4 late toxicities were observed in four patients (7%) and were symptomatic in three (5%).

The Centre de Protontherapie D'Orsay treated 45 patients to a median total dose delivered within the gross tumor volume of 67 (CGE) (range 60–70) (33). With a mean follow-up of 30.5 months, the 3-year local control rates for chordomas and chondrosarcomas were 83.1% and 90%, respectively, and 3-year overall survival rates were 91% and 90%, respectively. Young age at the time of radiotherapy

influenced local control positively ($P < 0.03$) in univariate analysis but not in multivariate analysis. Only two patients presented grade 3 or 4 complications. A further review of 67 patients (including some cervical spine) treated showed 3-year local control rates of 71% and 85% for chordomas and chondrosarcomas, respectively, and 3-year overall survival rates of 88% and 75%, respectively (34). Once again, on multivariate analysis, only age was an independent prognostic factor of local control.

The Paul Scherrer Institute treated 29 patients with chordomas and chondrosarcomas using spot-scanning proton radiotherapy to a median dose of 74 and 68 CGE, respectively (35). With a median follow-up of 29 months, the 3-year local control rates were 87.5% and 100% for chordoma and chondrosarcoma, respectively. At 3 years, actuarial progression-free survival and overall survival was 90% and 93.8%, respectively. Actuarial 3-year complication-free survival was 82.2%. Radiation-induced pituitary dysfunction was observed in 4 (14%) patients (CTCAE grade 2). No patient presented with postradiation brainstem or optic pathways necrosis or dysfunction. In univariate analysis, age ≤ 40 years at the time of proton therapy affected favorably on progression-free survival ($P = .09$). An update in 2009 showed an actuarial 5-year LC rate of 81% for chordomas and 94% for chondrosarcomas (36). Five-year rates of overall survival were 62% for chordomas and 91% for chondrosarcomas. High-grade late toxicity consisted of one patient with grade 3 and one patient with grade 4 unilateral optic neuropathy, and two patients with grade 3 CNS necrosis. No patient experienced brainstem toxicity. Actuarial 5-year freedom from high-grade toxicity was 94%. These results compare favorably to other combined proton-photon.

For all these institutions, the treatment of chordomas and chondrosarcomas remains to be a combination of both protons and photons. Torres et al (37) reviewed the "optimal treatment plan" for treatment of tumors located at the skull base. Five patients with skull base chordomas were used to generate four plans: an IMRT photon plan with a 1-mm planning target volume (PTV) for stereotactic treatment, an IMRT photon plan with a 3-mm PTV for standard treatment, a proton plan targeted at the clinical target volume (CTV), and a combination plan using the 3-mm PTV for photons and the CTV for protons. The primary objective was to achieve 95% or greater PTV-prescribed dose coverage. Proton plan was the least homogeneous and conformal. Dosimetric advantages were seen using either a 1-mm PTV for stereotactic treatment or a combined plan with this yielding the best target coverage and most conformality.

Consideration for the future will be assessment of neurocognitive function and fatigue levels in these patients as well as continuing to improve upon current treatment modalities including spot scanning.

Meningiomas

Meningiomas account for approximately 30% of primary intracranial neoplasms and are most commonly benign. Grade I meningiomas may be observed or treated with either surgical resection or SRS. However the rate of recurrence of grade II and III (atypical and malignant) meningiomas even after a complete surgical resection can be as high as 40% to 100% at 5 years (38). Photon therapy has been used to increase local control after surgical resection. The use of protons has been used for dose escalation particularly at the skull base where critical structures have historically prevented higher doses than 60 Gy.

Seventeen patients at the Centre de Protonthérapie d'Orsay with grades I to III meningiomas were treated with a combination of photons and proton therapy (39). The median total dose delivered was 61 CGE. With a median follow-up of 37 months, the 4-year local control and overall survival rates were 87.5 and 88.9, respectively. In South Africa, hypofractionated and SRS with protons was used to treat 27 patients with intracranial meningiomas (40). The mean dose for stereotactic treatment was 16.3 CGE and for the hypofractionated course was 61.6 CGE in 16 fractions.

Radiologic control was achieved in 88% of patients in the hypofractionated group and 100% in the stereotactic group. A total of three patients suffered permanent neurologic deficits (13%).

MGH published on 31 patients who underwent fractionated radiation therapy with either photons alone or in combination with protons (41). Target mean doses were 62 CGE (range 50–68) for atypical meningiomas and 58 CGE (range 40–72) for malignant meningiomas. The mean follow-up was 59 months. Actuarial local control rates at 8 years were similar for both histologies (19% for atypical and 17% for malignant). However, significantly improved local control was observed for proton versus photon radiation (80% versus 17% at 5 years, $P = 0.003$) and target doses ≥60 Gy for both atypical ($P = 0.025$) and malignant meningioma ($P = 0.0006$). Actuarial 8-year survival rate for malignant meningiomas was significantly improved by the use of proton over photon radiation and doses >60 CGE. Three patients developed symptomatic radiation damage after 59.3, 68.4, and 72 Gy/CGE. The Centre de Protonthérapie d'Orsay reviewed 24 patients with grade II and III meningiomas treated postoperatively with a combination of photon and proton radiotherapy (42). The mean total radiation dose was 65.01 CGE with a median follow-up of 32 months. The overall mean local relapse-free interval was 27.2 months (28.3 months for atypical meningioma and 23 months for malignant meningioma). The overall 8-year local control rate was 46.7% and the overall survival was 42.6%. Survival was significantly associated with total dose. There was no acute morbidity of radiotherapy. One patient developed radiation necrosis 16 months after treatment.

The PSI treated 16 patients with intracranial meningioma that was untreated, recurrent, or incompletely resected with a spot-scanning proton beam (43). The median prescribed dose was 56 CGE (range 52.2–64). With a median follow-up time of 34.1 months, the cumulative 3-year local control, progression-free survival, and overall survival were 91.7, 91.7, and 92.7%, respectively. No patient died from recurrent meningioma. Cumulative 3-year toxicity-free survival was 76.2%. One patient presented with radiation-induced optic neuropathy (SOMA grade 3) and retinopathy (SOMA grade 2) 8.8 and 30.4 months after treatment, respectively. These patients with ophthalmologic toxicity received doses higher than those allowed for the optic/ocular structures. Another patient developed a symptomatic brain necrosis (CTCAE grade 4) 7.2 months after treatment. No radiation-induced hypothalamic/pituitary dysfunction was observed.

Functional outcomes have also been followed in patients treated with a combination of photon and proton radiotherapy (44). Fifty-one patients with intracranial meningiomas of the base of the skull were treated with a median total dose was 60.6 CGE (range 54–64). The mean follow-up was 25.4 months. Acute tolerance was excellent. Out of the 108 eye-related symptoms, 106 (96%) were evaluated. Improvements were reported for 73 (68.8%) of them. Out of the 88 other miscellaneous symptoms, 81 (92%) were evaluated. Improvements were reported in 54 cases (67%). Median time to improvement ranged from 1 to 24 months after completion of the radiotherapy, depending on the symptom. Four-year local control and overall survival rates were 98% and 100%, respectively. Two patients complained of grade 3 side effects: one unilateral hearing loss requiring aid and one case of complete pituitary deficiency.

A retrospective review at MGH of 25 patients with optic nerve sheath meningiomas treated with conformal fractionated radiotherapy by either stereotactic photon or proton radiation was performed (45). The patients presented with symptoms of visual loss or orbital pain, or were incidentally diagnosed by imaging. The indication for treatment was the development or progression of symptoms. The median dose delivered was 50.4 CGE. At a median follow-up of 30 months, 95% had improved or stable visual acuity. One patient had worsened visual acuity after initial postirradiation improvement. Three patients had evidence of asymptomatic, limited retinopathy on ophthalmologic examination, and one had recurrent tumor 11 years after treatment.

Pituitary Adenomas

The role of proton therapy in both functioning and nonfunctioning pituitary adenomas continues to evolve as advances in megavoltage photons has made the dosimetric differences subtle. There are some limited data on proton therapy with a particular focus on functioning tumors as they typically require higher doses for control.

LLUMC published their series of 47 patients with pituitary adenomas treated with protons, who had at least 6 months of follow-up (46). Approximately half the tumors were functional. The median dose was 54 CGE in standard fractionation. Ninety-one percent had tumor stabilization as per follow-up imaging with 17 patients having functional adenomas that normalized or had decreased hormone levels. There was progression in three patients. Death was attributed to functional progression in two patients. Toxicity included temporal lobe necrosis (2%), new significant visual deficits in three patients (6%), and incident hypopituitarism (24%).

Proton stereotactic radiosurgery (PSR) has been delivered in patients with persistent acromegaly. Twenty-two patients were treated at MGH with a median dose of 20 CGE (range 15–24) (47). With a median follow-up of 6.3 years, a response was seen in 95% of patients, with 59% of patients having a complete response. No visual complications, seizures, clinical evidence of brain injury, or secondary tumors were noted. New pituitary deficits were seen in 38% of patients. The same group reviewed 38 patients with persistent Cushing's disease and Nelson's syndrome (48). Single-fraction PSR was delivered at a median dose of 20 CGE. At a median follow-up of 62 months, 100% of patients with Nelson's syndrome and 52% of patients with Cushing's disease achieved a complete response. The median time to a complete response was 18 months. No secondary tumors were noted on follow-up MRI scans, and there was no clinical evidence of optic nerve damage, seizure, or brain injury. Approximately half (52%) of patients developed new pituitary deficits.

Although promising, a review of the literature by the same group (49) shows that a direct comparison of clinical results attained using photon- and proton-based SRS are confounded by a bias toward reserving proton beams for the treatment of larger and more complex lesions. However, the physical properties of proton radiation offer superior conformality in dose distribution relative to photon irradiation, and this may be more apparent with the development of intensity-modulated proton techniques.

Craniopharyngioma

There are very limited data on the use of proton therapy for craniopharyngiomas. MGH has reviewed their series of 15 patients with craniopharyngioma who underwent combined proton and photon radiotherapy (50). The median dose prescribed to the tumor was 56.9 CGE (median proton component was 26.9 CGE). Median follow-up was 13.1 years. Actuarial 10-year survival rate was 72%. Actuarial 5- and 10-year local control rates were 93% and 85%, respectively. Results in terms of survival and local control are comparable with other contemporary series and although no formal neuropsychologic testing was performed, surrogate measures of lifestyle and professional accomplishments were within normal ranges.

Acoustic Neuromas/Vestibular Schwannomas

The treatment of acoustic neuromas has transitioned from surgery to radiation therapy particularly for small tumors amenable to radiosurgery. A recent review of the literature shows that the lack of uniform reporting criteria for tumor control, facial function and hearing preservation, and variability in follow-up times make it difficult to compare studies (and therefore treatment modalities γ-knife, linear accelerator, and proton beam) of radiation treatment for acoustic neuromas (51). LLUMC reviewed their series of 30 patients treated with proton beam

therapy who received 54.0 CGE in 30 fractions (patients with functional hearing) or 60.0 CGE in 30 to 33 fractions for patients without useful hearing (52). With a mean follow-up of 34 months, there was no evidence of disease progression. Of those patients with Gardner-Robertson grade I or II hearing, 31% maintained useful hearing. No transient or permanent treatment-related trigeminal or facial nerve dysfunction was observed.

MGH reviewed their series of patients who had undergone proton beam SRS (53). Sixty-eight patients were treated to a dose to the tumor margin (70% isodose line) of 12 Gy. At a mean clinical follow-up of 44 months, 54.7% were smaller and 39.1% were unchanged (tumor control rate 94%; actuarial control rate 94% at 2 years and 84% at 5 years). Three tumors enlarged. Three patients (4.7%) underwent shunting for hydrocephalus evident as increased ataxia. Of six patients with functional hearing ipsilaterally, one improved, one was unchanged, and four progressively lost hearing. Cranial neuropathies were infrequent: persistent facial hypesthesia (4.7%); intermittent facial paresthesias (9.4%); persistent facial weakness (4.7%) requiring oculoplasty; transient partial facial weakness (9.4%), and synkinesis (9.4%). More extensive review of 88 patients by Weber et al (54) showed actuarial 2- and 5-year tumor control rates of 95.3% and 93.6%. Of the 21 patients (24%) with functional hearing, 33.3% retained serviceable hearing ability. Actuarial 5-year normal facial and trigeminal nerve function preservation rates were 91.1% and 89.4%. Univariate analysis revealed that prescribed dose ($P = 0.005$), maximum dose ($P = 0.006$), and the inhomogeneity coefficient ($P = 0.03$) were associated with a significant risk of long-term facial neuropathy. No other cranial nerve deficits or cancer relapses were observed. Hypofractionation has also been used in larger acoustic neuromas (55). Fifty-one patients treated with hypofractionation (three fractions) to a mean dose of 26 CGE at the isocenter (mean minimum of 21.4 CGE) were followed for 72 months clinically and 60 months radiologically. The 5-year local control rate was 98%. Hearing preservation was seen in 42%, facial nerve preservation in 90.5%, and trigeminal nerve preservation in 93%.

■ TOXICITY IN BRAIN

Given the dosimetric properties of proton radiotherapy, there is a hypothesis that there will be less long-term side effects following proton radiotherapy than with photon radiotherapy. Given the small number of institutions that were using protons, conclusions were difficult to make. MGH published the long-term incidence of brainstem injury for their patients with chordomas and chondrosarcomas that were treated with a combination approach to total doses between 63 and 79.2 CGE (56). Doses to the brainstem surface were limited to ≤64 CGE and to the brainstem center to ≤53 CGE. With a mean follow-up of 42.5 months, actuarial rates of 5- and 10-year high-grade toxicity-free survival were 94% and 88%, respectively. Brainstem toxicity was observed in 17 patients (4.6%). Multivariate analysis

TABLE 1
Trials with Proton Therapy

Study	Institution	Title	Status
NCT01024907	UPenn	Proton beam radiation therapy in treating patients with low grade gliomas	Recruiting
NCT01063114	MGH/MDACC/NCI	Proton beam radiotherapy for medulloblastoma and pineoblastoma	Recruiting
NCT00105560	MGH/NCI	Proton beam radiation therapy in treating young patients who have undergone biopsy or surgery for medulloblastoma or pineoblastoma	Active, not recruiting
NCT01117844	UPenn	Proton radiation for meningomas and hemangiopericytomas	Recruiting
NCT01115777	MGH/MDACC	Prospective assessment of quality of life in pediatric patients treated with radiation therapy for brain tumors and non-CNS malignancies	Recruiting
NCT01067196	U Florida	Outcomes study of late effects after proton RT for CNS tumors in children	Recruiting
NCT00798057	U Florida	Proton radiation therapy for pituitary adenoma	Recruiting
NCT00496119	MDACC	Proton beam therapy for chordoma patients	Recruiting
NCT00496522	MDACC	Proton beam therapy for chondrosarcoma	Recruiting
NCT00797602	U Florida	Proton therapy for chordomas and/or chondrosarcomas outcomes protocol	Recruiting
NCT00713037	MGH	Hypoxia-positron emission tomography and intensity modulated proton therapy dose painting in patients with chordomas	Recruiting
NCT00592748	MGH	Charged particle RT for chordomas and chondrosarcomas of the base of skull or cervical spine	Active, not recruiting

Source: www.clinicaltrials.gov
Abbreviations: CNS, central nervous system; MDACC, M D Anderson Cancer Center; MGH, Massachusetts General Hospital; RT, radiotherapy; U Florida, University of Florida; UPenn, University of Pennsylvania.

identified three independent factors as important prognosticators for increased risk of brainstem toxicity: number of surgical procedures ($P < 0.001$), volume of the brainstem receiving 60 CGE ($P < 0.001$), and prevalence of diabetes ($P < 0.01$). This suggests that the tissue volume included in the high dose regions rather than the maximum dose of brainstem alone is significant when planning. In addition, predisposing factors and surgical manipulation contribute to the incidence of late effects. As with all radiation, risks have been reported. Chacko et al. (57) reported two cases of optic nerve complications following proton beam radiation therapy. The first patient received radiation after surgery for a clival chordoma and developed sequential radiation optic neuropathy at 5 and 9 months. The second patient developed optic nerve hemorrhage postradiotherapy for optic nerve sheath meningioma. Also important will be the rate of secondary malignancy following proton radiotherapy given the decrease in integral dose to the surrounding tissue. There has been evidence of an anaplastic glioma after proton beam radiotherapy treatment for a low-grade skull base chondrosarcoma (58). These usually occur 10 to 15 years after radiotherapy.

■ FUTURE

Current trials for protons in the treatment of brain tumors are growing given the number of locations now opening with protons. Table 1 summarizes current trials open and those for which we are awaiting results. Given the high cost for this modality (59), we will need to rely on these and other multi-institutional studies to guide us toward selecting the appropriate modality for each tumor type and, more importantly, each patient.

■ REFERENCES

1. American Cancer Society. *Cancer Facts & Figures 2010*. Atlanta, GA: American Cancer Society; 2010. http://www.cancer.org/Research/CancerFactsFigures/CancerFactsFigures/ACSPC-024113.

2. Stupp R, Mason WP, van den Bent MJ, et al. Radiotherapy plus concomitant and adjuvant temozolomide for glioblastoma. *N Engl J Med*. 2005;352 (10):987–996.

3. Mirimanoff RO, Gorlia T, Mason W, et al. Radiotherapy and temozolomide for newly diagnosed glioblastoma: recursive partitioning analysis of the EORTC 26981/22981-NCIC CE3 phase III randomized trial. *J Clin Oncol*. 2006;24(16):2563–2569.

4. Stratton K, Anderson A, Koehler AM. Effects of radiation mediating agents on the response of a murine ependymoma to proton irradiation. *Radiology*. 1966;87(1):68–73.

5. Nyström SH. Some aspects of the use of protons in the treatment of experimental brain tumors. *Naturwissenschaften*. 1966;53(6):159–160.

6. Nyström SH. Effects of high energy protons on brain and glioma of mice. *Acta Radiol Ther Phys Biol*. 1966;3:133–148.

7. Proton radiation for acromegaly. *N Engl J Med*. 1968; 278(13):732.

8. Kjellberg RN, Shintani A, Frantz AG, Kliman B. Proton-beam therapy in acromegaly. *N Engl J Med*. 1968;278(13):689–695.

9. Steward VW, Koehler AM. Proton radiography of a human brain tumor within the skull: a preliminary report. *Surg Neurol*. 1974;2(4):283–284.

10. Graffman S, Haymaker W, Hugosson R, Jung B. High-energy protons in the postoperative treatment of malignant glioma. *Acta Radiol Ther Phys Biol*. 1975; 14(5):443–461.

11. Kjellberg RN. Stereotactic Bragg peak proton beam radiosurgery for cerebral arteriovenous malformations. *Ann Clin Res*. 1986;18(suppl 47):17–19.

12. Barker FG 2nd, Butler WE, Lyons S, et al. Dose-volume prediction of radiation-related complications after proton beam radiosurgery for cerebral arteriovenous malformations. *J Neurosurg*. 2003;99(2):254–263.

13. Silander H, Pellettieri L, Enblad P, et al. Fractionated, stereotactic proton beam treatment of cerebral arteriovenous malformations. *Acta Neurol Scand*. 2004; 109(2):85–90.

14. Vernimmen FJ, Slabbert JP, Wilson JA, Fredericks S, Melvill R. Stereotactic proton beam therapy for intracranial arteriovenous malformations. *Int J Radiat Oncol Biol Phys*. 2005;62(1):44–52.

15. Hermanto U, Frija EK, Lii MJ, Chang EL, Mahajan A, Woo SY. Intensity-modulated radiotherapy (IMRT) and conventional three-dimensional conformal radiotherapy for high-grade gliomas: does IMRT increase

the integral dose to normal brain? *Int J Radiat Oncol Biol Phys*. 2007;67(4):1135–1144.

16. Zach L, Stall B, Ning H, et al. A dosimetric comparison of four treatment planning methods for high grade glioma. *Radiat Oncol*. 2009;4:45.

17. Chang EL, Wefel JS, Maor MH, et al. A pilot study of neurocognitive function in patients with one to three new brain metastases initially treated with stereotactic radiosurgery alone. *Neurosurgery*. 2007;60(2):277–83; discussion 283.

18. Merchant TE, Hua CH, Shukla H, Ying X, Nill S, Oelfke U. Proton versus photon radiotherapy for common pediatric brain tumors: comparison of models of dose characteristics and their relationship to cognitive function. *Pediatr Blood Cancer*. 2008;51(1):110–117.

19. Hug EB, Muenter MW, Archambeau JO, et al. Conformal proton radiation therapy for pediatric low-grade astrocytomas. *Strahlenther Onkol*. 2002; 178(1):10–17.

20. McAllister B, Archambeau JO, Nguyen MC, et al. Proton therapy for pediatric cranial tumors: preliminary report on treatment and disease-related morbidities. *Int J Radiat Oncol Biol Phys*. 1997;39(2):455–460.

21. Timmermann B, Lomax AJ, Nobile L, et al. Novel technique of craniospinal axis proton therapy with the spot-scanning system: avoidance of patching multiple fields and optimized ventral dose distribution. *Strahlenther Onkol*. 2007;183(12):685–688.

22. Fitzek MM, Thornton AF, Harsh G 4th, et al. Dose-escalation with proton/photon irradiation for Daumas-Duport lower-grade glioma: results of an institutional phase I/II trial. *Int J Radiat Oncol Biol Phys*. 2001;51(1):131–137.

23. Kelly PJ, Daumas-Duport C, Scheithauer BW, Kall BA, Kispert DB. Stereotactic histologic correlations of computed tomography- and magnetic resonance imaging-defined abnormalities in patients with glial neoplasms. *Mayo Clin Proc*. 1987;62(6):450–459.

24. Earnest F 4th, Kelly PJ, Scheithauer BW, et al. Cerebral astrocytomas: histopathologic correlation of MR and CT contrast enhancement with stereotactic biopsy. *Radiology*. 1988;166(3):823–827.

25. Tsien C, Moughan J, Michalski JM, et al.; Radiation Therapy Oncology Group Trial 98–03. Phase I three-dimensional conformal radiation dose escalation study in newly diagnosed glioblastoma: Radiation Therapy Oncology Group Trial 98–03. *Int J Radiat Oncol Biol Phys*. 2009;73(3):699–708.

26. Mizumoto M, Tsuboi K, Igaki H, et al. Phase I/II trial of hyperfractionated concomitant boost proton radiotherapy for supratentorial glioblastoma multiforme. *Int J Radiat Oncol Biol Phys*. 2010;77(1):98–105.

27. Nishizaki T, Saito K, Jimi Y, et al. The role of cyberknife radiosurgery/radiotherapy for brain metastases of multiple or large-size tumors. *Minim Invasive Neurosurg*. 2006;49(4):203–209.

28. Suit HD, Goitein M, Munzenrider J, et al. Definitive radiation therapy for chordoma and chondrosarcoma of base of skull and cervical spine. *J Neurosurg*. 1982;56(3):377–385.

29. Austin-Seymour M, Munzenrider J, Goitein M, et al. Fractionated proton radiation therapy of chordoma and low-grade chondrosarcoma of the base of the skull. *J Neurosurg*. 1989;70(1):13–17.

30. Santoni R, Liebsch N, Finkelstein DM, et al. Temporal lobe (TL) damage following surgery and high-dose photon and proton irradiation in 96 patients affected by chordomas and chondrosarcomas of the base of the skull. *Int J Radiat Oncol Biol Phys*. 1998;41(1): 59–68.

31. Munzenrider JE, Liebsch NJ. Proton therapy for tumors of the skull base. *Strahlenther Onkol*. 1999;175(suppl 2):57–63.

32. Hug EB, Loredo LN, Slater JD, et al. Proton radiation therapy for chordomas and chondrosarcomas of the skull base. *J Neurosurg*. 1999;91(3):432–439.

33. Noël G, Habrand JL, Mammar H, et al. Combination of photon and proton radiation therapy for chordomas and chondrosarcomas of the skull base: the Centre de Protonthérapie D'Orsay experience. *Int J Radiat Oncol Biol Phys*. 2001;51(2):392–398.

34. Noël G, Habrand JL, Jauffret E, et al. Radiation therapy for chordoma and chondrosarcoma of the skull base and the cervical spine. Prognostic factors and patterns of failure. *Strahlenther Onkol*. 2003;179(4): 241–248.

35. Weber DC, Rutz HP, Pedroni ES, et al. Results of spot-scanning proton radiation therapy for chordoma and chondrosarcoma of the skull base: the Paul Scherrer Institut experience. *Int J Radiat Oncol Biol Phys*. 2005;63(2):401–409.

36. Ares C, Hug EB, Lomax AJ, et al. Effectiveness and safety of spot scanning proton radiation therapy for chordomas and chondrosarcomas of the skull base: first long-term report. *Int J Radiat Oncol Biol Phys*. 2009;75(4):1111–1118.

37. Torres MA, Chang EL, Mahajan A, et al. Optimal treatment planning for skull base chordoma: photons, protons, or a combination of both? *Int J Radiat Oncol Biol Phys*. 2009;74(4):1033–1039.

38. Dziuk TW, Woo S, Butler EB, et al. Malignant meningioma: an indication for initial aggressive surgery and adjuvant radiotherapy. *J Neurooncol.* 1998;37(2):177–188.

39. Noël G, Habrand JL, Mammar H, et al. Highly conformal therapy using proton component in the management of meningiomas. Preliminary experience of the Centre de Protonthérapie d'Orsay. *Strahlenther Onkol.* 2002;178(9):480–485.

40. Vernimmen FJ, Harris JK, Wilson JA, Melvill R, Smit BJ, Slabbert JP. Stereotactic proton beam therapy of skull base meningiomas. *Int J Radiat Oncol Biol Phys.* 2001;49(1):99–105.

41. Hug EB, Devries A, Thornton AF, et al. Management of atypical and malignant meningiomas: role of high-dose, 3D-conformal radiation therapy. *J Neurooncol.* 2000;48(2):151–160.

42. Boskos C, Feuvret L, Noel G, et al. Combined proton and photon conformal radiotherapy for intracranial atypical and malignant meningioma. *Int J Radiat Oncol Biol Phys.* 2009;75(2):399–406.

43. Weber DC, Lomax AJ, Rutz HP, et al.; Swiss Proton Users Group. Spot-scanning proton radiation therapy for recurrent, residual or untreated intracranial meningiomas. *Radiother Oncol.* 2004;71(3):251–258.

44. Noël G, Bollet MA, Calugaru V, et al. Functional outcome of patients with benign meningioma treated by 3D conformal irradiation with a combination of photons and protons. *Int J Radiat Oncol Biol Phys.* 2005; 62(5):1412–1422.

45. Arvold ND, Lessell S, Bussiere M, et al. Visual outcome and tumor control after conformal radiotherapy for patients with optic nerve sheath meningioma. *Int J Radiat Oncol Biol Phys.* 2009;75(4):1166–1172.

46. Ronson BB, Schulte RW, Han KP, Loredo LN, Slater JM, Slater JD. Fractionated proton beam irradiation of pituitary adenomas. *Int J Radiat Oncol Biol Phys.* 2006; 64(2):425–434.

47. Petit JH, Biller BM, Coen JJ, et al. Proton stereotactic radiosurgery in management of persistent acromegaly. *Endocr Pract.* 2007;13(7):726–734.

48. Petit JH, Biller BM, Yock TI, et al. Proton stereotactic radiotherapy for persistent adrenocorticotropin-producing adenomas. *J Clin Endocrinol Metab.* 2008; 93(2):393–399.

49. Chen CC, Chapman P, Petit J, Loeffler J. Proton radiosurgery in neurosurgery. *Neurosurg Focus.* 2007; 23(6):E5.

50. Fitzek MM, Linggood RM, Adams J, Munzenrider JE. Combined proton and photon irradiation for craniopharyngioma: long-term results of the early cohort of patients treated at Harvard Cyclotron Laboratory and Massachusetts General Hospital. *Int J Radiat Oncol Biol Phys.* 2006;64(5):1348–1354.

51. Bassim MK, Berliner KI, Fisher LM, Brackmann DE, Friedman RA. Radiation therapy for the treatment of vestibular schwannoma: a critical evaluation of the state of the literature. *Otol Neurotol.* 2010;31(4):567–573.

52. Bush DA, McAllister CJ, Loredo LN, Johnson WD, Slater JM, Slater JD. Fractionated proton beam radiotherapy for acoustic neuroma. *Neurosurgery.* 2002; 50(2):270–3; discussion 273.

53. Harsh GR, Thornton AF, Chapman PH, Bussiere MR, Rabinov JD, Loeffler JS. Proton beam stereotactic radiosurgery of vestibular schwannomas. *Int J Radiat Oncol Biol Phys.* 2002;54(1):35–44.

54. Weber DC, Chan AW, Bussiere MR, et al. Proton beam radiosurgery for vestibular schwannoma: tumor control and cranial nerve toxicity. *Neurosurgery.* 2003; 53(3):577–86; discussion 586.

55. Vernimmen FJ, Mohamed Z, Slabbert JP, Wilson J. Long-term results of stereotactic proton beam radiotherapy for acoustic neuromas. *Radiother Oncol.* 2009; 90(2):208–212.

56. Debus J, Hug EB, Liebsch NJ, et al. Brainstem tolerance to conformal radiotherapy of skull base tumors. *Int J Radiat Oncol Biol Phys.* 1997;39(5):967–975.

57. Chacko JG, Schatz NJ, Glaser JS. Delayed optic nerve complications after proton beam irradiation. *Ann Ophthalmol (Skokie).* 2008;40(3–4):166–170.

58. Ehsani S, Hodaie M, Liebsch NJ, Gentili F, Kiehl TR. Anaplastic glioma after high-dose proton-photon radiation treatment for low-grade skull base chondrosarcoma. *J Neurooncol.* 2008;88(2):231–236.

59. Dvorak T, Wazer DE. Evaluation of potential proton therapy utilization in a market-based environment. *J Am Coll Radiol.* 2010;7(7):522–528.

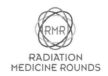

RADIATION
MEDICINE ROUNDS

Proton Therapy in Lung Cancer and Other Thoracic Tumors

Joe Y. Chang* and Ritsuko Komaki

The University of Texas MD Anderson Cancer Center, Houston, TX

■ ABSTRACT

Both lung and esophageal cancers are challenging diseases to treat. Radiation dose escalation/acceleration improves local control but also increases toxicity. Compared with photons, proton therapy spares more critical structures due to unique physical characteristics. By modulating the Bragg peak of protons in energy and time, a conformal radiation dose with or without intensity modulation can be delivered to the target while sparing the surrounding normal tissues. Thus, proton therapy is ideal when organ preservation is a priority. However, proton is more sensitive to organ motion and anatomy changes compared with photons. In this article, we review the practical issues of proton therapy, describe its image-guided treatment planning and delivery, discuss clinical outcomes for patients with non–small cell lung cancer and esophageal cancer who received this therapy, and suggest the challenges and future development of proton therapy.

Keywords: proton therapy, lung cancer, 4-D CT planning, adaptive radiotherapy, passive scattering proton therapy, scanning beam proton therapy

■ INTRODUCTON

Radiation therapy plays an essential role in the management of non–small cell lung cancer (NSCLC). Lung cancer is the cause of most cancer-related deaths and is associated with a 5-year overall survival rate of only 15% (1). For the past 3 decades, the "standard" treatment for inoperable stages I, II, or III NSCLC has been conventional photon radiotherapy, at a dose of 60 to 66 Gy delivered in 30 to 33 fractions (2). However, this regimen is associated with a local control of only 30% to 50% (2–5), and thus a more effective treatment is urgently needed.

Increasing clinical evidence suggests that in NSCLC there is a radiation dose-response

*Corresponding author, Department of Radiation Oncology, Unit 97, The University of Texas MD Anderson Cancer Center, 1515 Holcombe Blvd., Houston, TX 77030

E-mail address: jychang@mdanderson.org

Radiation Medicine Rounds 1:3 (2010) 523–538.
DOI: 10.5003/2151–4208.1.3.523

relationship that affects both overall survival and local control rates, with higher doses associated with better outcomes (6–8). However, higher radiation doses, particularly with concurrent chemotherapy, are associated with higher levels of toxicity (9). Three-dimensional conformal radiotherapy (3D-CRT) (10,11) and recently, stereotactic body radiation therapy (SBRT) (12–16), intensity-modulated radiation therapy (IMRT) (17,18), and proton therapy (19–21) using dose-escalated treatment appear to be alternatives to improve control of local disease and possibly overall survival rates with reduced toxicity in NSCLC.

Although 3D-CRT and IMRT have the potential to reduce toxicity to normal tissues, the relatively high exit dose from photon x-ray therapy limits the possibility of dose escalation or acceleration (15,18). A proton beam, on the other hand, is made up of charged particles (protons) that have a well-defined range of penetration into tissue (22). As the proton beam penetrates the body, its particles slow down and deposit a large portion of their energy near the end of their range. The resulting central axis depth dose distribution is known as the Bragg peak (22). By modulating the Bragg peak in both energy and time, a full, localized, and uniform dose can be delivered to the target while sparing the surrounding normal tissue (22–24). Thus, proton therapy is ideal when organ preservation is a priority, particularly in patients with lung (24) and esophageal cancers (25).

Esophageal cancer is the seventh leading cause of cancer deaths worldwide (1). While squamous cell carcinoma is the most prevalent histology in the world, adenocarcinoma of the distal esophagus accounts for nearly 50% of cases in developed countries. While surgery is the mainstay of treatment of esophageal cancer, the use of chemoradiation—postoperatively, neoadjuvantly, or definitively—has become standard practice in the United States. The pathologic complete response (pCR) rate for preoperative chemoradiation is about 25% to 40% (26–28). There has been significant improvement in the overall survival rate and median survival rate for patients treated with preoperative chemoradiotherapy compared with surgery alone, particularly for patients with pCR (26–28). Although radiation dose escalation may potentially increase pCR rate, preoperative chemoradiation is associated with higher postoperative mortality rate (26–28). For patients who received definitive chemoradiotherapy without surgery, about one fifth were cured, as demonstrated by the Radiation Therapy Oncology group 8501 (29). It is no coincidence that the pCR rate is also around 25% after preoperative chemoradiation, and studies have demonstrated that pCR is one of the strongest predictors of long-term survival after preoperative chemoradiation (30). Therefore, further reducing the normal tissue dose may reduce postoperative mortality, improve pCR rates, and allow dose escalation in definitive treatment. Proton therapy may help to achieve these goals (25).

Despite decades of clinical experience, knowledge of proton therapy is still basic, and many questions remain unanswered, particularly concerning the effect of tumor motion during and between treatments (22,23,31–33). Thus, there are many opportunities to improve the distribution of proton doses, including the use of intensity-modulated proton therapy (IMPT) (34,35), stereotactic body proton therapy (SBPT), (36) and image-guided interventions for both interfractional and intrafractional variations (22,23,31–33). Such techniques have the potential to reduce uncertainties and improve therapeutic potential of proton therapy.

■ PRACTICAL ISSUES OF PROTON THERAPY

Treatment Planning for Passively Scattered Proton Therapy

Several differences exist between proton and photon treatment planning (22–24). First, changing the patient's position as a whole along the path of the beam has virtually no effect on proton dose distribution, whereas tissue variation in the proton's path due to intrafractional or interfractional motion and anatomic changes (such as tumor shrinkage, weight loss, and lung inflammation or consolidation) may affect the range of the protons (31–33).

Second, the concept of the planning target volume (PTV) margin typically used in photon therapy (i.e., uniform and 3D expansion from clinical target volume (CTV) to create PTV margin) is inapplicable to proton therapy. Photons have only lateral edges, and therefore the PTV margin is fixed based on setup uncertainty and motion. In contrast, proton beams essentially have three edges: the two lateral penumbras resulting from coulomb multiple scattering and the distal edge. Also, the depth dependence of the lateral penumbras in the proton beam is stronger than that of photon for depths more than about 17 cm; for shallower depths, the proton lateral penumbra is generally smaller than that of the photon. In general, each proton treatment beam must have its own distal and proximal margins that depend on the distance traveled by the beam in the tissue (23). Therefore, uniformly expanding the CTV to the PTV is not valid. However, the magnitude of lateral margins may be determined using the same method as that used for the CTV-to-PTV margin for photons (23,24).

Third, "smearing" the compensator is another strategy to ensure coverage of the target in proton therapy in the presence of motion and variations of structures normal to the beam direction (23). Smearing compensates for possible small misalignment of the compensator with the patient's anatomy due to changes in anatomy or positioning uncertainties. The smearing process essentially reduces the width of higher-thickness regions of the compensator to allow protons to penetrate deeper, even when adjacent higher-density tissues move into its path. This parameter is user controlled and can be adjusted during planning. Smearing the compensator and including margins for range uncertainty ensures coverage of the target at the expense of delivering a higher dose of protons to normal tissue distal to the target (23).

Four-dimensional computed tomographic (4D-CT) scans that comprise multiple 3D-CTs in a

sequence of phases of the respiratory cycle are being used in planning both photon-based and proton-based treatments that include a motion-integrated internal target volume (ITV) enveloping the moving target (37). Due to the considerable impact of motion in proton dose distribution, 4D-CT–based simulation is highly recommended for proton planning (31,32). To design the compensator for proton-based treatment, the density at each point in the ITV should be set to the maximal density in any one of the phases, not to the average density of all phases (32). This strategy ensures that protons will penetrate deep enough to adequately cover the target, regardless of its position (32). The treatment plan should still be calculated in an averaged CT database using ITV density override (see next section for details).

In the overall treatment-planning process for a specified beam direction, a typical proton treatment-planning system first determines the maximal water equivalent (WE) thickness depth of penetration to the distal edge of the target plus the margin and the minimal WE depth to the target minus the margin (23). These quantities are then used to determine the range, and therefore the energy, of incident protons and the width of the spread-out Bragg peak (SOBP). The range and SOBP are eventually used to select parameters for treatment machines (e.g., range-modulation wheel, second scatterer, energy range shifters) required for delivering the proton beam. For each beam, the proton treatment-planning system also creates a block conforming to the beam's eye view shape of the CTV plus appropriate margins for setup and motion uncertainties normal to the beam direction and for the beam penumbra. Dose distributions for each beam are then calculated and summed for plan evaluation (23).

As with x-ray and electron treatments, proton treatments use multiple fields (often noncoplanar) to keep the skin dose to reasonable limits and to spare normal tissues in the beam path (23,24). However, as mentioned previously, treatment-planning strategies involving protons can be quite different from those involving x-rays and electrons because of the particular properties of proton beams. For example, in proton-based treatments, the rapid distal falloff of the proton dose distribution permits the planner to aim a proton beam directly at a critical normal structure, compared with x-ray–based and electron-based therapies, which may deliver a toxic dose to critical structures distal to the target because of the higher exit dose. However, there is uncertainty about the travel range of protons in the body and about the possible increased relative biologic effectiveness (RBE) toward the end of the SOBP. Therefore, caution should be observed because of the behavioral interactions of the protons in the body and because of the various uncertainties encountered in this type of therapy.

As mentioned previously, motion and interfractional changes in inhomogeneous structures in the path of protons also affect the range of protons (31–33). The uncertainty about proton range may also be associated with the correlation between CT Hounsfield units and the proton mass stopping power of tissues (38,39). This uncertainty has a negligible effect on photon dose distributions; however, the uncertainty about proton range effects much more importantly because of the protons' charge, weight, and manner of scattering (38,39). This factor affecting the range of protons is that the transport of protons through complex inhomogeneities, such as those encountered in the lung, degrades the proton range; protons do not stop at a sharp edge as they would in homogeneous material. Range uncertainties can result in the proton beam stopping prematurely, the target being underdosed, or the beam extending beyond the target and possibly overdosing critical structures. Such concerns are particularly important for low-density regions around lung and esophageal tumors. A correlation between CT Hounsfield units and proton mass stopping powers, based on measurements of materials of known stopping powers on the CT scanner, is used to calculate proton ranges in tissue (38,39). However, the issue of reducing the uncertainty associated with CT Hounsfield units and proton mass stopping powers still needs to be addressed.

The advantages of passive scattering systems include their safety, simplicity, and lower sensitivity to the time structure of the accelerator. Although these systems have well served their intended purpose, passive scattering systems have a number of disadvantages, the most serious of which being that they are only about 20% to 40% efficient and therefore waste a large number of protons in the scattering system and in the beam-limiting aperture. This substantial loss of protons can pose a problem for synchrotron-based proton therapy systems, in which the dose rate is more limited than that in cyclotrons. Passive scattering systems also tend to be sensitive to variations in the beam position. Furthermore, when protons are stopped in the scattering system and aperture, they produce secondary neutrons, many of which can contribute to the whole-body dose to the patient (40). Neutrons have a high RBE and are believed to be the source of secondary cancers in some patients (40). However, matched study to compare the secondary malignancy in patients who received either proton therapy or photon therapy showed that passive scattering proton therapy (PSPT) still reduced the secondary malignancy from 12% of photon to 6.4 % of proton (41).

Another disadvantage of the passive scattering system is that it produces a single SOBP for the entire target volume; thus, during treatment of large irregular target volumes with notable differences in their thickest and thinnest depths, the high-dose region needs to be pulled back to avoid overdosing distal critical structures while target volume with thicker depth will be underdosing or covers the target volume with thickest depth but overdosing critical structures. Therefore, this system may not be an ideal approach for tumors with complicated anatomy such as lesions curved around critical structures (34,36). IMPT will resolve these issues as described in the following section (34,36).

Dynamic Spot Scanning and IMPT

In dynamic spot scanning, the Bragg peak of a narrow pencil beam entering the treatment nozzle is magnetically scanned across the target cross section, and the energy of the protons is adjusted to vary the depth of the spot to achieve the intended dose pattern (42). The beam can be either scanned continuously in a raster scan pattern or stopped at discrete, predetermined positions for a specified time to deliver the desired dose (42).

In discrete spot scanning, the beam is turned off during travel between the spots (42–45). The deepest layer of tumor is scanned by selecting the appropriate energy; when scanning of that layer is completed, the energy is decreased and the next layer is scanned. In this manner, the entire target volume can be irradiated either to deliver a uniform dose distribution for each field, much like the passive scattering method, or to deliver a nonuniform dose distribution for each field in such a way that when the doses from all the fields are summed, the total dose distribution is uniform. This process is called IMPT (42–44). To produce a nonuniform dose distribution with raster scanning, the intensity of the beam can be varied continuously as the spot is moved.

Dynamic spot scanning has several advantages: it provides full 3D shaping of the dose distribution to the target volume, no devices such as dose-limiting apertures or range compensators are required, the efficiency is high because very few protons are wasted, and very few neutrons are produced (40). One disadvantage of dynamic spot scanning is the difficulty in delivering a desired dose to tumors that move during irradiation. For the proton scanning beam approach, such as the approach used in IMPT, treatment delivery with active beam scanning introduces the problem of interplay effects when the pencil beam moves on a time scale similar to that of intrafractional tumor motion (43).

In situations where fractionation may not provide enough repetition to blur the interplay effects, repeated delivery or "repainting" of each field several times within a fraction has been suggested (43). Beam-gating techniques such as respiratory-gated or breath-hold proton beam radiotherapies should decrease the uncertainty in such treatments.

Although proton therapy is very precise with sharp edges, the uncertainty of motion and density change remain to be addressed, particularly the use of IMPT in lung cancer.

IMPT plans are optimized with an "inverse" treatment-planning system that is similar to the inverse planning for IMRT (42–44). However, IMPT has an additional degree of freedom because the energy of each proton pencil beam, in addition to its intensity, can be varied, which increases the dose-shaping potential of IMPT. Although IMPT and IMRT have equally complex treatment plans, the IMPT plans will always be superior to IMRT plans due to the Bragg peak, especially in the sparing of normal tissue (34,35). On average, IMPT uses half the integral dose used by IMRT, resulting in substantial sparing of critical tissues and organs (35). The coverage of the target volume, however, can be quite similar for both IMPT and IMRT.

■ RBE OF PROTON THERAPY

Clinically Used RBE and Potential Uncertainty

Proton beams are essentially a form of low linear energy transfer radiation. Protons have nearly the same RBE as do photons. However, the RBE of a proton beam depends on tissue type, dose, dose rate, energy, and depth of penetration (46). Paganetti et al. (46) summarized findings from numerous experiments with protons and concluded that the RBE of protons is approximately 1.1; an RBE of 1.1 is considered standard in routine clinical practice. The computed physical dose distribution is multiplied by the RBE to obtain the cobalt gray equivalent (CGE) or Gy (RBE) dose distribution.

However, the RBE has been shown to vary with the linear energy transfer, which increases as the energy of protons decreases with increasing depth of penetration (46). This effect may be particularly pronounced near the end of the proton range. This variation in RBE is typically ignored, and the biologically effective dose near the end of the range is likely to be higher than that seen in a treatment plan. For this reason and because of uncertainties in range, aiming the beams toward a normal critical structure in very close proximity to the target should be avoided, particularly when the number of beams in the treatment plan is small.

Treatment resistance caused by cancer stem cells (CSCs) is a challenging clinical issue. Targeting CSCs may improve cancer cure rate. The RBE of protons is assumed to be close to that of photons at 1.1 as mentioned earlier. However, the tissue- and cell-specific RBEs and the molecular mechanisms of proton therapy in treatment-resistant cancer cells such as CSCs are not well understood. A recent study indicated that protons might be more effective than photons are in eliminating treatment-resistant CSCs in vitro (47). Additional study is needed to validate this finding in the clinical setting.

■ CONSIDERATION OF 4D-CT–BASED TUMOR MOTION

As discussed previously, proton therapy is very sensitive to motion and tissue density changes, so proper management of tumor motion reduces underdosing of the target and overdosing of normal tissues. The development of multislice detectors and faster imaging reconstruction has enabled real-time imaging of patients and the assessment of organ motion using 4D-CT (48).

4D-CT images can also be used to delineate internal gross tumor volume (IGTV), which envelops the GTV motion throughout the respiratory cycle (37). Delineating the IGTV from 4D-CT images involves outlining the tumor volume on the expiratory-phase images and then registering the outline to the images from other phases to create a union of target contours enclosing all possible positions of the target. Another method of defining the IGTV is to create a maximum intensity projection (MIP) image by combining data from the multiple CT data sets with data from the respiratory cycle and modifying the IGTV by visually verifying the target volume throughout all (typically 10) breathing phases (37). Relying on the MIP image alone, without modifying the tumor volume across the breathing phases, may cause target volume underestimation, especially for lesions near the diaphragm, chest wall, and mediastinal structures (49). In the treatment-planning process that uses ITV, IGTV is first created with MIP for the compensator design (32). This IGTV MIP approach achieved dose distributions similar to those actually delivered to patients over the course of proton therapy (32). Compared with the approach that uses a large smearing margin in highly mobile lung tumors, as proposed by Moyers et al. (23), the IGTV MIP approach achieves similar target coverage while sparing more normal tissue because a universally large smearing margin is not used (32). Instead, an individualized IGTV based on actual tumor motion is used for the compensator design. Although this approach may slightly overtreat the normal tissues behind the tumor when the tumor moves out of the field, it does ensure that the whole tumor is treated adequately no matter where it moves during the different phases of breathing.

To evaluate the impact of tumor motion and strategy to address the motion issue in esophageal cancer, we studied the impact of selecting different data sets from 4D-CT imaging during proton treatment planning in patients with distal esophageal cancer. The effects of changes in 4D-CT data set and smearing margins in proton treatment planning for five patients with distal esophageal cancer whose diaphragms were in the beam path and could move several centimeters during respiration were analyzed (50). The result showed that using the inspiration CT plus a smearing margin can lead to adequate ICTV coverage in treatment plans for patients with distal esophageal tumors surrounded by tissue that is subject to large changes in density during a proton treatment. More studies are needed to validate our observations.

■ IMAGE-GUIDED DELIVERY OF ADAPTIVE PROTON THERAPY

Interfractional tumor motion and anatomic changes during radiation therapy are major causes of target miss and/or overtreating normal tissues in lung cancer. As a result of these issues, an initial simulation-based treatment plan may not match the treatment delivered, particularly for proton therapy. Weekly 4D CT study was conducted to investigate the magnitude of the changes in tumor volume and mobility in NSCLC during 7 weeks of radiotherapy (51). Tumor volume reduction ranged from 20% to 71% and tumor mobility significantly increased. In some cases, an explicit initial determination of the IGTV may not be sufficient to cover the target, owing to variations in tumor motion and anatomy during treatment. Insufficiency of the IGTV coverage was even more severe with significant tumor underdosing in selective cases when proton treatment was used (33). Proton has been shown to be more sensitive in motion/anatomy change than IMRT over 7 weeks of radiotherapy. Replanning of radiotherapy using repeat 4D CT images to adapt to changes in patient anatomy and organ motion between treatment fractions might be warranted for selective highly mobile tumors to reduce the potential for missing the target and/or overdosing the normal tissues during proton therapy (Figure 1).

■ PROTON-IMPROVED SPARING OF NORMAL TISSUE

Virtual Clinical Trial Comparing Proton Therapy, 3D-CRT, and IMRT

In 2006, a virtual clinical trial was conducted in patients with either stage I or stage IIIA/B NSCLC to compare dose-volume histograms for those treated with standard-dose 3D-CRT or IMRT with histograms of patients treated with simple passive scattering 3D (without IMPT) proton radiotherapy at standard or escalated doses (24). Compared with standard-dose (60–66 Gy) photon therapy, proton treatment statistically significantly reduced the dose to normal tissues including the lungs, esophagus, spinal cord, and heart, even with dose escalation. The improvement was even more

Photon 3-DCRT	Proton

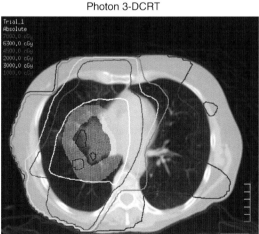 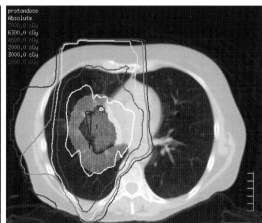

FIGURE 1
Comparison of photon three-dimensional conformal radiotherapy with passive scattering proton therapy in stage III non–small cell lung cancer.

Before RT   3 weeks during RT

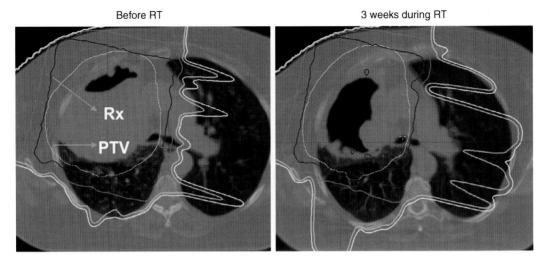

FIGURE 2
Change of tumor size/density during 7 weeks of radiotherapy impacts the length of proton path and justifies adaptive replanning in stage III non–small cell lung cancer.

dramatic in the sparing of the heart, spinal cord, and normal lung low-dose exposure at dose of 5 Gy (V5, see Figure 2). In addition, proton therapy caused a 33% to 60% rate of absolute improvement of the nontarget integral dose. Findings from this trial indicated that proton therapy with dose escalation and/or acceleration (74 Gy for stage III and 87.5 Gy for stage I NSCLC) may translate to better local control and survival rates that are achieved with standard doses of photon therapy without increasing the toxicity in patients with NSCLC.

Since the study findings were published, IMRT techniques in lung cancer have been improved clinically. More clinical experience using IMRT in lung cancer resulted in the development of an optimized IMRT autoplan system at The University of Texas MD Anderson Cancer Center. A virtual clinical study showed significant improvement of sparing of normal tissue compared with a previous version of the IMRT planning algorithm (Unpublished data). Our laboratory then reanalyzed the previously reported cases and compared current optimized IMRT with PSPT. We found that low-dose (V5) exposure of protons still spared

substantially more heart, spinal cord, and lung tissue, in addition to reducing the nontarget integral dose. However, the advantage of sparing lung volume receiving a dose ≥20 Gy using proton therapy compared with photon therapy was no longer seen due to limited proton beam numbers and angles. Optimized proton therapy, such as IMPT, is needed in future studies to address these issues.

To explore the proton therapy in distal esophageal cancer, we conducted a virtual clinical study in 15 patients with distal esophageal cancer (25) to compare 3D and 4D CT-based treatment plans for proton therapy or IMRT for esophageal cancer and examined doses to the lung, heart, and spinal cord and variations in target coverage and normal tissue sparing. The results showed that, compared with IMRT, median lung volumes exposed to 5, 10, and 20 Gy and mean lung doses were reduced significantly. The greater lung sparing in the two-beam proton plan was achieved at the expense of less conformity to the target and greater irradiation of the heart compared with the IMRT plan or the three-beam proton plan. The difference in spinal cord maximum dose between

3D and 4D plans could exceed 5 Gy for the proton plans, partly owing to variations in filling of stomach gas (25). Proton therapy provided significantly better sparing of lung than did IMRT. Motion of the diaphragm and filling of stomach gas must be considered when evaluating target coverage and spinal cord doses.

Although PSPT appears to be promising in reducing toxic effects of radiation therapy, physicians are also facing a clinical challenge with dose-escalated radiotherapy using PSPT for lung tumors in very complicated cases such as contralateral hilar or supraclavicular lymph node involvement, or tumors adjacent to the esophagus and spinal cord (34). Because of a limited number of treatment fields, it is very difficult to use PSPT to deliver ablative doses to targets with complicated shapes or locations, such as tumors curved around sensitive critical structures. In such cases, compromised dose coverage has to be considered to avoid damaging critical normal tissue structures (34).

Unlike PSPT, IMPT using scanning beam therapy can simultaneously optimize the intensities and energies of all pencil beams using an objective function that accounts for targets as well as normal tissue constraints (34). To compare IMPT with IMRT and PSPT for stage IIIB NSCLC with complicated anatomy and to explore the possibility of individualized radical radiotherapy, we conducted a virtual clinical study to deliver IMRT at 63 Gy, PSPT at 74 Gy, and IMPT at the same doses of 63 Gy, 74 Gy, and individualized highest dose of radical radiotherapy possibly achieved without beyond maximal tolerable dose (MTD) (34). Compared with IMRT, IMPT spared more lung, heart, spinal cord, and esophagus tissue, even with dose escalation from 63 Gy to 83.5 Gy with a mean MTD of 74 Gy. Compared with PSPT, IMPT allowed further dose escalation from 74 Gy with a mean MTD of 84.4 Gy (range, 79.4–88.4 Gy) while keeping all parameters of normal tissue sparing lower or similar to that of PSPT. In addition, IMPT prevented lower target coverage in patients with complicated tumor anatomies. IMPT further reduces the dose for normal tissue

and allows individualized radical radiotherapy for extensive stage IIIB NSCLC.

SBRT is emerging as a standard treatment for inoperable stage I NSCLC with local control rates typically exceeding 90% (12–16). However, using SBRT for patients with tumors located centrally or superiorly in the lung and/or near critical structures (e.g., major pulmonary vessels, spinal cord, esophagus, or bronchial tree) is particularly challenging due to the potential complications from radiation-induced damage to these critical structures (15). To minimize toxicity while maintaining tumor coverage with SBRT for centrally or superiorly located stage I NSCLC, we investigated PSPT and IMPT (36). Our data showed that for centrally or superiorly located stage I NSCLC, proton therapy (particularly IMPT) delivered ablative doses to the target volume and significantly reduced doses to the surrounding normal tissues compared with that of photon SBRT.

Clinical Treatment Outcome

Several clinical trials have studied patients with NSCLC who underwent proton radiotherapy (52–56). These clinical trials focused on dose-escalated or accelerated proton therapy in early-stage disease and showed promising clinical results.

Shioyama et al. (52) reported the clinical outcome of 28 patients with stage I NSCLC treated with proton radiotherapy to median total dose of 76 Gy (RBE) (range, 49–93 Gy [RBE]) in a median of 3-Gy (RBE) fractions (range, 2–6 Gy [RBE]). The 5-year overall survival rate was 70%, with a local control rate of 89% for patients with stage IA (<3 cm) disease. However, the local control rate for patients with larger tumors (stage IB) was considerably lower at 39%, indicating that higher radiation doses were needed. Recurrence in the mediastinum was reported in 21% of the cases, and the 5-year overall survival rate was 15%. Only one case of grade 3 acute toxicity and no severe late toxicity was observed. Because a positron emission tomographic (PET) scan was not used for clinical staging in this study, it is possible that the stage IB cases had been understaged, particularly with regard to disease in the mediastinal lymph nodes.

In another study of proton radiotherapy for stage I NSCLC, Bush et al. (53) treated 68 patients with proton therapy (total dose of 60–70 Gy [RBE] in 10 fractions). This regimen resulted in a local control rate of 87% in T1 lesions and 49% in T2 lesions; the 3-year disease-free survival rate was 72%. No patients developed G2 or above pneumonitis or esophagitis. Hata et al. (54) reported preliminary results of a study of hypofractionated proton therapy for 21 patients with stage I NSCLC (tumors <4.2 cm); a dose of 50 to 60 Gy was given in 10 fractions. Local progression-free and disease-free rates were 95% and 79% at 2 years, respectively, with no grade 3 or higher toxicities.

In a similar study, Nihei et al. (55) used proton therapy to treat 36 patients with stage I NSCLC using a total dose of 70 to 94 CGE delivered in 20 fractions and found similarly high rates of local control (92.6%) and overall survival (81%) at 2 years. No grade 2 or higher acute toxicity was observed, but late grade 3 toxicity was observed in three patients. Among the 19 patients with stage IB disease, two had local progression and eight developed regional lymph node or distant metastasis.

Nakayama et al. (56) used proton therapy to treat 55 medically inoperable patients with stage I NSCLC using a total dose of 66 GyE in 10 fractions for peripherally located tumors and 72.6 GyE in 22 fractions for centrally located tumors. The overall and progression-free survival and tumor local control rates at 2 years were 97.8%, 88.7%, and 97.0%. Two patients (3.6%) had deterioration in pulmonary function, and two patients (3.6%) had grade 3 pneumonitis.

Recent meta-analysis indicated that survival rates for particle therapy such as proton were higher than those for 3D-CRT, but similar to SBRT in stage I inoperable NSCLC. Proton therapy may be more beneficial in stage III NSCLC, especially in reducing adverse events (57). These clinical studies showed the safety and efficacy of proton therapy in early-stage NSCLC. However, the optimal regimen of proton therapy has not been well defined. In most studies, the doses were low compared with the current standard. In addition, simple 3D proton therapy was used in these studies; optimized proton therapy such as respiratory-gated therapy was not available, and image-guided radiotherapy was not strictly applied.

To analyze the toxicity and patterns of failure of proton therapy given in ablative doses for medically inoperable T1N0M0 (central location) or T2–3N0M0 (any location) NSCLC, we conducted a phase I/II study at MD Anderson Cancer Center to deliver 87.5 Gy (RBE) at 2.5 Gy/fraction (19). All patients underwent treatment simulation with 4D-CT; IGTVs were delineated on MIP images and modified by visual verification of the target volume in 10 breathing phases. The IGTV with MIP density was used to design compensators and apertures to account for tumor motion. Therapy consisted of passively scattered protons, and all patients underwent repeat 4D-CT simulations during treatment to assess the need for adaptive replanning. At a median follow-up time of 16.3 months (range, 4.8–36.3 months), no patient had experienced grades 4 or 5 of toxicity. The most common adverse effect was dermatitis (grade 2, 67%; grade 3, 17%), followed by grade 2 fatigue (44%), grade 2 pneumonitis (11%), grade 2 esophagitis (6%), and grade 2 chest wall pain (6%). Rates of local control were 88.9%, regional lymph node failure was 11.1%, and distant metastasis was 27.8%. Twelve patients (67%) were still alive at the last follow-up; five had died of metastatic disease and one of a preexisting cardiac disease.

Our study showed that ablative doses of proton therapy can be safely delivered to targets with a large tumor size and/or challenging location with minimal toxicity using image-guided adaptive proton therapy in early-stage NSCLC (19). Compared with most of the previous studies, patients in our study had larger tumor sizes and/or more challenging tumor locations. The ablative doses (biologic effective dose, RBE > 100 Gy) that we delivered to the targets were higher than those in the literature and achieved promising local control with minimal toxicity.

These previous findings (19,52–56) suggest that passively scattered proton therapy has the potential to deliver ablative radiation doses with little toxicity in early-stage lung cancer. Additional improvements in conformality for cases involving complicated anatomy, such as tumors that curve around sensitive critical structures, can be achieved by IMPT (58). Our findings from our phase-I study support the validity of conducting a phase II study using this approach; such a trial is currently being conducted at MD Anderson Cancer Center and Massachusetts General Hospital.

Minimal clinical data are available about proton therapy for patients with stage III NSCLC, the most common stage requiring radiotherapy. MD Anderson Cancer Center analyzed patterns of failure, survival, and toxicity for patients with stage III NSCLC treated with dose-escalated (74 CGE) proton therapy with concurrent chemotherapy in our phase II clinical study (20,21). Most patients were not considered good candidates for the conventional dose (63 Gy) using photon therapy due to bulky primary, contralateral mediastinum/hilum and/or supraclavicular lymph node involvement. All patients underwent PET/CT staging and 4D-CT simulation-based treatment planning and adaptive proton delivery. With a median follow-up of 16 months (range, 7–26 months), no patients had experienced grade 4 or 5 toxicity. The most common nonhematologic grade 3 adverse effect was dermatitis (13.3%), followed by esophagitis (6.7%) and pneumonitis (3.3%). Rate of isolated local failure within planned target volume was 13.3%, rate of regional lymph node failure outside planned target volume was 13.3%, rate of distant metastasis was 20%, and rate of combined distant metastasis and local/regional failure was 16.7%. Compared with our historical clinical outcomes using IMRT in stage IIII NSCLC, proton therapy appears to significantly reduce side effects, particularly for pneumonitis and esophagitis. Dose-escalated concurrent proton therapy and chemotherapy appear to improve local control and reduce toxicity. Additional studies are needed to address the issues of missing targets and treatment uncertainty using proton therapy. Longer follow-up time is also needed. Optimization of proton therapy with the appropriate management of uncertainties is actively being investigated. Image-guided respiratory-gated proton therapy and IMPT will be implemented in the near future (58).

To address the efficacy and toxicity of proton therapy compared with IMRT in NSCLC, supported by National Institutes of Health program grant, MD Anderson Cancer Center and Massachusetts General Hospital are conducting randomized studies to compare IMRT with proton therapy using 74 Gy with concurrent chemotherapy in stage III NSCLC. In addition, image-guided stereotactic hypofractionated proton radiotherapy will be implemented for patients with early-stage NSCLC and results will be compared with hypofractionated stereotactic photon-based body radiotherapy, particularly for those with centrally located early-stage NSCLC.

For esophageal cancer, a clinical study of patients with locally advanced squamous cell carcinoma treated with combined photon and proton therapy without chemotherapy at a dose of 76 to 82 Gy (range, 69.1–89.5 Gy) showed 5-year actuarial survival rates for the 46 patients, patients with T1 (n = 23), and those with T2–T4 (n = 23) of 34%, 55%, and 13%, respectively (59). The 5-year disease-specific survival rates for the 46 patients, those with T1, and those with T2–T4 were 67%, 95%, and 33%, respectively. The 5-year local control rates for patients with T1 and T2–T4 lesions were 83% and 29%, respectively. Concurrent chemoradiotherapy using proton therapy showed promising outcomes with reduced toxicity (60).

■ SUMMARY AND FUTURE DEVELOPMENT

The dose distributions of proton Bragg peaks led to the development of proton therapy that was superior to photon therapy for reducing the radiation dose to normal tissue adjacent to the target, such as esophagus, lung, heart, and spinal cord tissues, and also to intervening tissues in the path of the radiation beams. However, planning and delivery of image-guided proton therapy are crucial to appropriately manage uncertainties induced by anatomic variations and by organ or tumor motions.

Reduced tumor motion is required for optimal image-guided proton therapy. 4D-CT planning is recommended for all proton therapy, particularly for IMPT. Respiratory-gated proton treatment further improves normal tissue sparing. More efficient CT imaging that will be performed before each proton therapy treatment is being developed and will facilitate greater accuracy in treatment delivery. Resimulation during treatment is recommended for selected patients with substantial tumor shrinkage and possible lung expansion.

Because of the reductions in the "dose bath" and in the volume of normal tissues irradiated with proton therapy, patients' tolerance of radiation and/or chemoradiotherapy would be enhanced, thus allowing higher doses of these treatments to be delivered. Delivery of higher proton therapy doses, combined with the increased accuracy obtained from image-guided targeting and greater avoidance of normal tissues, would lead to reduced toxicity and better local disease control and survival rates in patients with NSCLC.

Compared with photon IMRT or SBRT, proton-based IMPT and SBPT achieve better target coverage and remarkable normal tissue sparing, particularly in clinically challenging cases. However, before IMPT is used in clinical settings, particularly for hypofractionated stereotactic treatment, more studies are needed to validate the impact of these uncertainties, since small lesions could move more significantly and there is less chance of averaged out uncertainty due to a lower fraction number. In addition, most proton therapy facilities only have on-board kilo-voltage x-ray imaging but lack volumetric imaging such as cone-beam CT or CT-on-rail, which have been widely used in photon SBRT. Implanted fiducial markers to improve clinical setup and target verification, particularly for respiratory-gated treatment, may be needed. Alternatively, volumetric verification, either outside or inside the proton treatment room before each fraction of treatment, should be explored. The use of proton therapy (particularly IMPT) in a clinical setting may translate to better local control, better survival, and less toxicity in patients with NSCLC. Actual Clinical studies are needed to validate our virtual clinical data.

Proton therapy has the potential to spare more critical structures and allow dose escalation in esophageal cancer treatment. However, tumor motion may have significant impact on dose distribution. Additional studies, particularly clinical trials, are needed.

Based on preliminary data from lung cancer, we have started to treat other thoracic malignancies such as thymoma and lymphoma with proton therapy. It is anticipated that long-term toxicities such as heart damage and secondary malignancy may be significantly reduced for these groups of patients who have favorable long-term survival outcome.

■ ACKNOWLEDGMENT

Our research was supported in part by P01-CA021239 from the National Cancer Institute.

■ REFERENCES

1. Jemal A, Siegel R, Ward E, Hao Y, Xu J, Thun MJ. Cancer statistics, 2009. *CA Cancer J Clin.* 2009;59(4):225–249.
2. Perez CA, Stanley K, Grundy G, et al. Impact of irradiation technique and tumor extent in tumor control and survival of patients with unresectable non-oat cell carcinoma of the lung: report by the Radiation Therapy Oncology Group. *Cancer.* 1982;50(6):1091–1099.
3. Kaskowitz L, Graham MV, Emami B, Halverson KJ, Rush C. Radiation therapy alone for stage I non-small cell lung cancer. *Int J Radiat Oncol Biol Phys.* 1993;27(3):517–523.
4. Dosoretz DE, Katin MJ, Blitzer PH, et al. Medically inoperable lung carcinoma: the role of radiation therapy. *Semin Radiat Oncol.* 1996;6(2):98–104.

5. Dosoretz DE, Galmarini D, Rubenstein JH, et al. Local control in medically inoperable lung cancer: an analysis of its importance in outcome and factors determining the probability of tumor eradication. *Int J Radiat Oncol Biol Phys*. 1993;27(3):507–516.

6. Rosenman JG, Halle JS, Socinski MA, et al. High-dose conformal radiotherapy for treatment of stage IIIA/IIIB non-small-cell lung cancer: technical issues and results of a phase I/II trial. *Int J Radiat Oncol Biol Phys*. 2002;54(2):348–356.

7. Kong FM, Ten Haken RK, Schipper MJ, et al. High-dose radiation improved local tumor control and overall survival in patients with inoperable/unresectable non-small-cell lung cancer: long-term results of a radiation dose escalation study. *Int J Radiat Oncol Biol Phys*. 2005;63(2):324–333.

8. Choi NC, Doucette JA. Improved survival of patients with unresectable non-small-cell bronchogenic carcinoma by an innovated high-dose en-bloc radiotherapeutic approach. *Cancer*. 1981;48(1):101–109.

9. Curran W, Scott C, Langer C, et al. Long term benefit is observed in a phase III comparison of sequential vs concurrent chemo-radiation for patients with unresected stage III NSCLC: RTOG 9410. *Proc Am Soc Clin Oncol*. 2003;22:621.

10. Socinski MA, Rosenman JG, Halle J, et al. Dose-escalating conformal thoracic radiation therapy with induction and concurrent carboplatin/paclitaxel in unresectable stage IIIA/B nonsmall cell lung carcinoma: a modified phase I/II trial. *Cancer*. 2001;92(5):1213–1223.

11. Schild SE, McGinnis WL, Graham D, et al. Results of a Phase I trial of concurrent chemotherapy and escalating doses of radiation for unresectable non-small-cell lung cancer. *Int J Radiat Oncol Biol Phys*. 2006;65(4):1106–1111.

12. Xia T, Li H, Sun Q, et al. Promising clinical outcome of stereotactic body radiation therapy for patients with inoperable Stage I/II non-small-cell lung cancer. *Int J Radiat Oncol Biol Phys*. 2006;66(1):117–125.

13. Onishi H, Shirato H, Nagata Y, et al. Hypofractionated stereotactic radiotherapy (HypoFXSRT) for stage I non-small cell lung cancer: updated results of 257 patients in a Japanese multi-institutional study. *J Thorac Oncol*. 2007;2(7 suppl 3):S94–100.

14. Nagata Y, Takayama K, Matsuo Y, et al. Clinical outcomes of a phase I/II study of 48 Gy of stereotactic body radiotherapy in 4 fractions for primary lung cancer using a stereotactic body frame. *Int J Radiat Oncol Biol Phys*. 2005;63(5):1427–1431.

15. Timmerman R, McGarry R, Yiannoutsos C, et al. Excessive toxicity when treating central tumors in a phase II study of stereotactic body radiation therapy for medically inoperable early-stage lung cancer. *J Clin Oncol*. 2006;24(30):4833–4839.

16. Chang JY, Balter PA, Dong L, et al. Stereotactic body radiation therapy in centrally and superiorly located stage I or isolated recurrent non-small-cell lung cancer. *Int J Radiat Oncol Biol Phys*. 2008;72(4):967–971.

17. Yom SS, Liao Z, Liu HH, et al. Initial evaluation of treatment-related pneumonitis in advanced-stage non-small-cell lung cancer patients treated with concurrent chemotherapy and intensity-modulated radiotherapy. *Int J Radiat Oncol Biol Phys*. 2007;68(1):94–102.

18. Liao ZX, Komaki RR, Thames HD Jr, et al. Influence of technologic advances on outcomes in patients with unresectable, locally advanced non-small-cell lung cancer receiving concomitant chemoradiotherapy. *Int J Radiat Oncol Biol Phys*. 2010;76(3):775–781.

19. Chang JY, Komaki R, Wen HY, et al. Toxicity and Patterns of failure of adaptive/ablative proton therapy for early-stage, medically inoperable Non-Small Cell Lung Cancer. *Int J Radiat Oncol Biol Phys* 2010: In Press.

20. Cox JD, Chang JY, Liao Z, et al. Acute esophageal reactions from proton beam therapy and concurrent chemotherapy for NSCLC: reduction in incidence and severity despite higher doses. *J Thorac Oncol*. 2007;2:S449.

21. Chang JY, Komaki R, Bucci MK, et al. Failure patterns and toxicity of concurrent proton therapy and chemotherapy for Stage III Non-small Cell Lung Cancer. *Int J Rad Onc Bio Phy*. 2009;75(3):S446.

22. Goitein M, Lomax A, Pedroni E. Treating cancer with protons. *Phys Today*. 2002;55:45–50.

23. Moyers MF, Miller DW, Bush DA, Slater JD. Methodologies and tools for proton beam design for lung tumors. *Int J Radiat Oncol Biol Phys*. 2001;49(5):1429–1438.

24. Chang JY, Zhang X, Wang X, et al. Significant reduction of normal tissue dose by proton radiotherapy compared with three-dimensional conformal or intensity-modulated radiation therapy in Stage I or Stage III non-small-cell lung cancer. *Int J Radiat Oncol Biol Phys*. 2006;65(4):1087–1096.

25. Pan X, Zhang X, Li Y, Mohan R, Liao Z. Impact of using different four-dimensional computed tomography data sets to design proton treatment plans for distal esophageal cancer. *Int J Radiat Oncol Biol Phys*. 2009;73(2):601–609.

26. Walsh TN, Noonan N, Hollywood D, Kelly A, Keeling N, Hennessy TP. A comparison of multimodal therapy and surgery for esophageal adenocarcinoma. *N Engl J Med*. 1996;335(7):462–467.

27. Urba SG, Orringer MB, Turrisi A, Iannettoni M, Forastiere A, Strawderman M. Randomized trial of preoperative chemoradiation versus surgery alone in patients with locoregional esophageal carcinoma. *J Clin Oncol.* 2001;19(2):305–313.

28. Gebski V, Burmeister B, Smithers BM, Foo K, Zalcberg J, Simes J; Australasian Gastro-Intestinal Trials Group. Survival benefits from neoadjuvant chemoradiotherapy or chemotherapy in oesophageal carcinoma: a meta-analysis. *Lancet Oncol.* 2007;8(3):226–234.

29. Cooper JS, Guo MD, Herskovic A, et al. Chemoradiotherapy of locally advanced esophageal cancer: long-term follow-up of a prospective randomized trial (RTOG 85–01). Radiation Therapy Oncology Group. *JAMA.* 1999;281(17):1623–1627.

30. Rohatgi P, Swisher SG, Correa AM, et al. Characterization of pathologic complete response after preoperative chemoradiotherapy in carcinoma of the esophagus and outcome after pathologic complete response. *Cancer.* 2005;104(11):2365–2372.

31. Engelsman M, Rietzel E, Kooy HM. Four-dimensional proton treatment planning for lung tumors. *Int J Radiat Oncol Biol Phys.* 2006;64(5):1589–1595.

32. Kang Y, Zhang X, Chang JY, et al. 4D Proton treatment planning strategy for mobile lung tumors. *Int J Radiat Oncol Biol Phys.* 2007;67(3):906–914.

33. Hui Z, Zhang X, Starkschall G, et al. Effects of inter-fractional motion and anatomic changes on proton therapy dose distribution in lung cancer. *Int J Radiat Oncol Biol Phys.* 2008;72(5):1385–1395.

34. Zhang X, Li Y, Pan X, et al. Intensity-modulated proton therapy reduces normal tissue doses compared with intensity-modulated radiation therapy or passive scattering proton therapy and enables individualized radical radiotherapy for extensive stage IIIB non-small cell lung cancer: a virtual clinical study. *Int J Rad Oncol Biol Phys.* [In press, Epub ahead of print]

35. Lomax AJ, Bortfeld T, Goitein G, et al. A treatment planning inter-comparison of proton and intensity modulated photon radiotherapy. *Radiother Oncol.* 1999;51(3):257–271.

36. Register SP, Zhang X, Mohan R, Chang JY. Proton stereotactic body radiation therapy for clinically challenging cases of centrally and superiorly located stage I non-small-cell lung cancer. *Int J Radiat Oncol Biol Phys.* 2010. [Epub ahead of print].

37. Chang JY, Dong L, Liu H, et al. Image-guided radiation therapy for non-small cell lung cancer. *J Thorac Oncol.* 2008;3(2):177–186.

38. Schneider U, Pedroni E, Lomax A. The calibration of CT Hounsfield units for radiotherapy treatment planning. *Phys Med Biol.* 1996;41(1):111–124.

39. Kanematsu N, Matsufuji N, Kohno R, Minohara S, Kanai T. A CT calibration method based on the poly-binary tissue model for radiotherapy treatment planning. *Phys Med Biol.* 2003;48(8):1053–1064.

40. Hall EJ. Intensity-modulated radiation therapy, protons, and the risk of second cancers. *Int J Radiat Oncol Biol Phys.* 2006;65(1):1–7.

41. Chung CS, Keating N, Yock T, Tarbell N. Comparative analysis of second malignancy risk in patients treated with proton therapy versus conventional photon therapy. *J Radiat Oncol Biol Phys.* 2008; 72(1):S8.

42. Kanai T, Kawachi K, Kumamoto Y, et al. Spot scanning system for proton radiotherapy. *Med Phys.* 1980;7(4):365–369.

43. Seco J, Robertson D, Trofimov A, Paganetti H. Breathing interplay effects during proton beam scanning: simulation and statistical analysis. *Phys Med Biol.* 2009;54(14):N283–N294.

44. Oelfke U, Bortfeld T. Inverse planning for photon and proton beams. *Med Dosim.* 2001;26(2):113–124.

45. Bortfeld T. An analytical approximation of the Bragg curve for therapeutic proton beams. *Med Phys.* 1997;24(12):2024–2033.

46. Paganetti H, Niemierko A, Ancukiewicz M, et al. Relative biological effectiveness (RBE) values for proton beam therapy. *Int J Radiat Oncol Biol Phys.* 2002;53(2):407–421.

47. Chang JY, Zhang X, Feng B, et al. Proton therapy targets cancer stem cells in treatment-resistant non-small cell lung cancer. *Int J Radiat Oncol Biol Phys* 2010: In press.

48. Liu H, Balter P, Tutt T, et al. Assessing respiration-induced tumor motion and internal target volume using 4-D CT for radiation therapy of lung cancer. *Int J Radiat Oncol Biol Phys.* 2007;68:531–540.

49. Ezhil M, Vedam S, Balter P, et al. Determination of patient-specific internal gross tumor volumes for lung cancer using four-dimensional computed tomography. *Radiat Oncol.* 2009;4:4.

50. Zhang X, Zhao KL, Guerrero TM, et al. Four-dimensional computed tomography-based treatment planning for intensity-modulated radiation therapy and proton therapy for distal esophageal cancer. *Int J Radiat Oncol Biol Phys.* 2008;72(1):278–287.

51. Britton KR, Starkschall G, Tucker SL, et al. Assessment of gross tumor volume regression and motion changes

during radiotherapy for non-small-cell lung cancer as measured by four-dimensional computed tomography. *Int J Radiat Oncol Biol Phys.* 2007;68(4): 1036–1046.

52. Shioyama Y, Tokuuye K, Okumura T, et al. Clinical evaluation of proton radiotherapy for non-small-cell lung cancer. *Int J Radiat Oncol Biol Phys.* 2003; 56(1):7–13.

53. Bush DA, Slater JD, Shin BB, Cheek G, Miller DW, Slater JM. Hypofractionated proton beam radiotherapy for stage I lung cancer. *Chest.* 2004;126(4):1198–1203.

54. Hata M, Tokuuye K, Kagei K, et al. Hypofractionated high-dose proton beam therapy for stage I non-small-cell lung cancer: preliminary results of a phase I/II clinical study. *Int J Radiat Oncol Biol Phys.* 2007;68(3):786–793.

55. Nihei K, Ogino T, Ishikura S, Nishimura H. High-dose proton beam therapy for Stage I non-small-cell lung cancer. *Int J Radiat Oncol Biol Phys.* 2006; 65(1):107–111.

56. Nakayama H, Sugahara S, Tokita M, et al. Proton beam therapy for patients with medically inoperable stage I non-small-cell lung cancer at the university of tsukuba. *Int J Radiat Oncol Biol Phys.* 2010;78(2):467–471.

57. Grutters JP, Kessels AG, Pijls-Johannesma M, De Ruysscher D, Joore MA, Lambin P. Comparison of the effectiveness of radiotherapy with photons, protons and carbon-ions for non-small cell lung cancer: a meta-analysis. *Radiother Oncol.* 2010;95(1):32–40.

58. Chang JY, Cox JD. Improving radiation conformality in the treatment of non-small cell lung cancer. *Semin Radiat Oncol.* 2010;20(3):171–177.

59. Sugahara S, Tokuuye K, Okumura T, et al. Clinical results of proton beam therapy for cancer of the esophagus. *Int J Radiat Oncol Biol Phys.* 2005;61(1):76–84.

60. Xiaomao G, Liao ZX, Komaki R, et al. Concurrent chemotherapy and proton beam therapy for esophageal cancer. *Int J Radiat Oncol Biol Phys.* 2009;75(3):S289–S290.

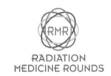

Proton Therapy: Project Planning and Development

Lynda J. Mischel*

University of Pennsylvania Health System, Philadelphia, PA

■ ABSTRACT

Investing and building a proton center requires significant planning and management. The planning a development may take more than 3 years and a wide range of resources. This paper presents an overview of the planning requirements for funding, vendor evaluation, operational structure and governance.

Keywords: Proton Center, business planning, governance

Developing a proton therapy center is a multi-year, resource intensive project. The clinical faculty of the Department of Radiation Oncology at Penn Medicine spent almost 10 years building a clinical plan and working with institutional leadership to develop a viable business model. That is not to suggest that a proton center needs to consume multiple years in development but to emphasize that this almost $200 million project is complex and must have significant clinical, financial, and institutional support in order to come to fruition. Many centers across the United States and globally have stalled in the development stage due to the sheer complexity of the project and a lack of required resources. However, a successful center can meet the needs of a broad population of patients, encourage academic research, and be financially successful.

The following will outline the overall planning and development requirements for a proton facility. Included are some of the research and development activities that we anticipate will be ongoing with the development of proton technology. Of course,

*Corresponding author, Department of Radiation Oncology, University of Pennsylvania Health System, Philadelphia, PA

E-mail address: Lynda.mischel@uphs.upenn.edu

Radiation Medicine Rounds 1:3 (2010) 539–544.
DOI: 10.5003/2151–4208.1.3.539

each individual institution will have its own set of requirements as reflected in the Roberts Proton Center at Penn Medicine. The Penn Center is committed to treating a broad range of patients and supporting the academic career of our faculty. To this end, we are implementing, in partnership with our vendors, four modalities of treatment, have developed a multi-leaf collimator for our gantries, and are pushing forward the complexity of clinical care offered to our patients. We are also committed to the integration of clinical care with conventional radiation as well as medical and surgical oncology.

■ CAPITAL PLANNING

A complete capital plan includes all of the equipment, building, and land necessary to open a proton facility. The first step in any business planning function is to develop an analysis of the "barriers to entry." For proton centers, the largest barrier is access to the necessary capital to build and operate a multiroom proton center. Many institutions will wait for the development of a less expensive single room option rather than take on the $150 to $200 million cost of a four to five room center. The return on investment analysis should be carefully considered with realistic operating assumptions for any of these options.

As an institution begins the capital planning process for a multiroom center, the following capital options may be explored:

- Institutional operating capital
- Debt funding
- Partnerships with local and regional institutions
- Philanthropy
- Partnership with a proton development company

■ BUSINESS PLANNING

The first phase of the business planning process will lead to the ultimate "go" or "no go" decision.

Each of the following steps is a necessary part of the decision-making process.

Facility Planning and Development

Identification of the appropriate facility site is an obvious first step to the facility planning process. The site considerations include building size (most proton facilities are upward of 60,000 square feet), as well as appropriate parking for patients, physicians, and staff. The gantries require at least a three-story height clearance for development. At Penn, we decided early in the process to integrate the proton treatment and research area with the conventional radiation department and maintain close proximity to the Abramson Cancer Center. This allowed some integration of the clinical and support staff as well as encouraged medical and surgical oncologists to participate in the early planning phases. We also built the proton center in close proximity to the Children's Hospital of Philadelphia, one of our capital partners and important patient base.

The cost of land development ranges dramatically across the country and may be important in choosing an equipment vendor. The building and land development constraints should be part of the information available in the equipment vetting process.

Operating Model

Building a realistic operating model is an essential part of the decision-making process. The model should include:

- Gross and net revenue assumptions
- Volume assumptions
- Ramp-up or carrying period costs
- Operating costs
- Staffing and training
- Marketing
- Contingency costs

Revenue

Rate determination is the most institutional specific part of the modeling process. To date, each Medicare carrier has a different policy regarding disease site-specific benefits; moreover, CMS has not made a formal coverage determination. Several of the large national insurance providers have published proton-specific coverage policies; some have restrictions on disease site. Local carriers, including the Blues, have vastly different coverage and benefit policies. Many regional and local carriers have not developed any policy and are making patient-specific decisions about coverage. Each institution will need to review revenue assumptions with institutional or local managed care specialists. The decisions made by these organizations have caused marked differences in net revenue per patient across the country.

As with rate modeling, each institution needs to develop a volume model to determine not only revenue but ultimately staffing requirements as well. We have seen many institutions use very aggressive volume assumptions to present an extremely aggressive ROI analysis. In general, each additional treatment room will become available for patient use every 3 months following acceptance of the first room. Institutions are working on decreasing the acceptance and commissioning schedule, but this remains a challenge. We have also found that during the acceptance period, many centers have had unexpected delays. If research and development activities are part of the project, some delays should be built into the ramp-up schedule.

We have found that treatment time is about 20% to 40% longer than conventional treatment regardless of disease site. One approach to volume modeling that does not require predicting disease mix is to use an average conventional treatment time and gross up by 30% to 40%. Another approach is to develop a disease site ramp-up plan, which allows more predictability in patient mix, but may be more difficult to implement as patients present for evaluation.

Start-Up Costs

During the development or ramp-up period, the vast majority of costs are in staff, recruitment, and training for both physicians and physicists. At Penn, we developed a weeklong training class for all of our integrated physician and physics staff. Many of our clinical team also traveled extensively to PTCOG educational and scientific programs, as well as other proton centers to learn from others in the field.

Other costs included travel to vendor facilities to monitor progress and QI procedures as well as to work through issues as they arose. This period of the project is much more time consuming than expected and may require several physics and physician full-time employees as well as a full-time project manager.

Operating Model

The vast majority of operating costs will involve staffing and training. Penn used staffing ratios similar to the conventional staffing for radiation therapy, nursing, social work, and other clinical support staff. As other institutions will attest, the staffing for dosimetry and physics is significantly more than needed in a photon setting.

The recruitment, onboarding and training costs for all of these new staff is also significant. Our model includes 3 months of training for all clinical staff, but we have found that treatment planning needs more intensive training. Six months is the current plan.

An expanded clinical research team has also been required at Penn. Establishing and managing clinical protocol development has far exceeded our experience in photons. Patient management, education, and protocol compliance are significant and require additional staff.

Fortunately, the integrated model at Penn allowed the management team already in place to contribute to the operating model. Without an existing management structure in place, a new center would need to plan for the hiring of this team 12 months prior to first patient.

The business office and intake staff also needs to be in place at least 3 months prior to opening. Payor education and rate negotiation should begin 18 months prior to opening in order to develop needed business office functions. Patients began calling for protons almost a full year prior to the go-live date. These costs were integrated into the existing operation but should be considered for a freestanding proton center.

Physician services modeling may take several forms; at Penn all of the physicians are employed by the University and have academic, teaching, and clinical responsibilities. Therefore, salaries were modeled using the structure used for all department physicians. In centers that will partner with physicians, a model needs to be developed based on expected volumes and incentives.

Support staff, including environmental services, maintenance, security, and so on, needs consideration for cost modeling as well. Information systems and technology support needs to be robust and may be the highest cost in this category.

The marketing and advertising budget needs to be reviewed by experts in the field. These costs are generally much higher than those of us with clinical management expertise expect but are a necessary part of opening a new center.

Finally, a placeholder in the operating model for contingency expenses protects the plan from unexpected delays or changes in insurance reimbursement. Many models exist for contingency planning; however using a percentage of net patient revenue is a simple and straightforward approach.

■ EQUIPMENT AND VENDOR CHOICE

Choosing a vendor for proton equipment, a treatment planning system, and an oncology information system will take from 12 to 24 months. Each system has benefits and limitations as does each company. These are some important issues for consideration when choosing proton delivery equipment:

- Clinical flexibility
- Operational up-time guarantees
- Service expectations
- Secure commitment to long-term clinical research and development
- Integration capabilities
- Proven timeliness
- Financial security

As with any new technology, the field will grow and change with unexpected speed. All systems will need to be able to adapt to clinical research developments and technological advances.

Treatment planning and OIS system companies also need to be able to make similar commitments to ongoing research and development, flexibility, and financial security. Moreover, these systems should be able to integrate with some proton delivery system. Many institutions are treating patients that require several modalities for treatment and the ability for the systems to integrate is a great advantage. Integrated systems also lead to more flexibility if and when the proton system has down time. Patients may be transferred to intensity-modulated radiation therapy with relative ease using the same system. Penn has used this integration to our patients benefit several times during the acceptance and commissioning phase of the project.

Imaging equipment is also a necessary consideration for future proton or photon centers. Positron emission tomography, magnetic resonance imaging, and computed tomography simulation are available and should be considered during the planning phase. The differences in imaging and simulations need to be reviewed by the clinical leadership and a facility and operation plan developed for the use of this equipment. Academic institutions should also consider the research requirements with the use of multiple imaging systems.

Contracting

Good legal advice and negotiation management is an essential part to executing a successful proton therapy center. The legal management team will likely need to negotiate and coordinate contracts with several equipment vendors as well as general contractors and possibly physicians simultaneously. Each contract needs a solid set of incentives and penalties so that all of the stakeholders are incented to work together when issues arise. The equipment contracts should address the following issues:

- Room delivery schedule
- Specifications for all modalities of equipment
- Schedule of payments
- Incentives and penalties
- Building specifications
- Change order system

Academic institutions will also need to address issues of intellectual property when research and development contracts are considered.

■ GOVERNANCE AND PROJECT MANAGEMENT

Once an institution has committed to developing a proton center, full-time, experienced project management is essential to the success of the program. The project manager is responsible for understanding and managing all of the points of intersection in the project plan. Whether the new center is free standing or in a large academic center, management of all of the work among the stakeholders is essential. Initially, the project manager will work with vendors to assure that the project adheres to the schedule and any building issues are addressed in a timely fashion. The project manager should also develop a regular reporting system so that all of the stakeholders have a regular update.

Following delivery of the initial equipment, the new site will take on a great deal of activity. The vendor staff and center staff will begin to interact on a daily basis. Keep in mind that the onsite team not only includes vendors and physics staff but also a construction team. Here, the project manager can help the on-site team develop a working relationship and work with leaders from all participants to ease the inevitable site difficulties. Some other responsibilities of the project manager may include:

- Contract and payment management
- Purchasing
- Change order process
- Communication among vendors and contractors
- Special projects
- Reporting

The project manager will also be responsible to educate the new management team about the complexities of the project and stakeholders. In many circumstances, the new management team will take over direct responsibilities of the project manager.

Governance

Any project of this size will have competing needs and necessitate management of ongoing training. To balance all of the competing requirements and continue to resource the projects requirements, the proton center will need a governance committee very early in the process. The membership of this group should represent all stakeholders at the highest level. Our executive committee included physician, physics, business, and administrative representatives.

The governance committee will need to be prepared to make decision regarding major changes in the project schedule, equipment availability, and financial management. This team will also be responsible for communicating with other members of the community about the benefits of the proton center. At Penn, members of this team worked with institution-managed care staff to educate local and regional payers, participated in the development of marketing and public relations plans, developed resources to educate the broader medical community, and supported the development of clinical research protocols. Ultimately, this team must also evaluate, manage, and support the necessary resources to make the proton center successful.

■ CONCLUSION

A proton therapy center may be the largest single clinical investment that an institution will make. It will take 3 to 5 years to bring to fruition and will test the resolve of all of the stakeholders at some point during the project. Each step in the project planning process requires concentrated effort. The resources necessary are great. However, if managed well, an institution and members of the team will develop clinical and research programs that will benefit a broad range of patients throughout the community and the institution itself.

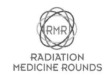

Proton Therapy in the Community

Sameer Keole

Oklahoma University Health Science Center, Oklahoma City, OK

■ **ABSTRACT**

Interest in proton therapy (PT) is increasing within the field of radiation oncology. Recent developments have allowed the implementation of PT into community settings. Large community-based radiation oncology practices may have the resources required to safely implement this new technology, especially if choosing the right partners. It is unlikely that widespread proliferation of PT will occur in the next decade, due to the complexity of projects. Community-based PT programs are able to contribute to the scientific advancement of particle therapy by participating and enrolling patients on clinical studies. The addition of new PT companies will also likely increase competition, driving down costs while improving the technology.

Keywords: proton therapy, proton, radiation oncology

On August 24, 2009, an Oklahoma man with a brain tumor began a curative intent course of external-beam radiation therapy (EBRT). This was unique in that the radiation modality was protons and the setting was a community practice.

We believe that this is the first time proton therapy has been used outside the walls of an "academic" institution. To some, this might raise several questions:

1. How did proton therapy end up in community-based radiation oncology practice in Oklahoma?
2. Can proton therapy be delivered in the community setting?

*Corresponding author, Adjunct Assistant Professor, Department of Radiation Oncology, Oklahoma University Health Science Center, Oklahoma City, OK
   E-mail address: sameer.keole@okc.procure.com

Radiation Medicine Rounds 1:3 (2010) 545–554.
DOI: 10.5003/2151–4208.1.3.545

demosmedpub.com/rmr

3. Will the use of proton therapy rise exponentially in the next decade, much like intensity-modulated radiation therapy (IMRT) in the previous decade?
4. What will be the impact of for-profit companies in proton therapy?
5. In an area of radiation oncology, which requires additional data, can a community practice contribute to answer questions?
6. Can a community practice treat the rare and complicated cases such as pediatric tumors?
7. What, if anything, has been learned in Oklahoma since last August regarding proton therapy?

■ WHY PROTONS IN OKLAHOMA?

In 2005, the founding members of Radiation Medicine Associates (RMA), a community-based radiation oncology practice in Oklahoma decided to explore the possibility of adding proton therapy to its practice. Members of the group had been among the first practitioners in the country to treat with IMRT (in 1993) and were early adopters of other treatment techniques such as prostate brachytherapy and Gamma Knife radiosurgery. They felt as though x-ray therapy, while still incredibly effective, was fast approaching its technical limits and that proton therapy offered a superior treatment option for a significant number of their patients. They also realized that bringing proton therapy into their own practice, without outside assistance, would be impossible. All of these issues led RMA to partner with a "third party" vendor (ProCure Treatment Systems), which could help them with financing, choosing a hospital partner, building the facility, and running the daily technical operations, without giving up medical decision-making within the center. By April 2007, full financing had been obtained, a hospital partner had been chosen, and thus a groundbreaking was held to begin construction on the ProCure Proton Therapy Center (PPTC) in Oklahoma City. Twenty-eight months later, the first patient was treated. This timeline is much shorter, by several years, than any other operational proton center in the United States, if not the world.

■ CAN PROTONS BE DELIVERED IN THE COMMUNITY SETTING?

A community radiation oncology group can successfully implement proton therapy into their practice—if the right partners are chosen. It is not practical to expect any group of physicians, much less than those in a busy clinical practice, to oversee aspects of financing, building construction, equipment installation, proton commissioning, and finally day-to-day facility management. Beyond this is the issue of proton therapy training.

Training is a major component of being prepared to treat patients in a safe and efficient manner from the opening of any new radiation center, proton or x-ray. Experience from several centers spanning decades have proven protons are not experimental and can be delivered safely (1,2). But even these centers were not able to simulate treating patients with proton therapy before actually doing it; instead, the training was often "on-the-job." Prior to the opening of the PPTC, new proton centers would send faculty to currently operating proton centers (such as MGH or Loma Linda) to observe treatments and interact with staff at those facilities. Although such trips were useful, they lacked structure and there was no ability to "educate" the trainees because the clinic environment was live. In 2007, ProCure Treatment Systems opened the Training and Development Center (TDC) in Bloomington, IN. The TDC is a 15,000 sq ft facility designed to be "Proton Therapy University."

The TDC is designed to mimic a proton treatment room at any ProCure facility in the country (currently, additional ProCure facilities are under construction in Illinois and New Jersey). Everything required for a proton treatment is in place—except the cyclotron. There are two treatment rooms, one with a gantry and one with an inclined beam line arrangement. Both rooms are equipped with on-board imaging (OBI) capabilities. This equipment (manufactured by Ion Beam Applications [IBA]) is identical to the equipment in the PPTC Oklahoma. The robotic patients positioning systems are also identical between the TDC and the PPTC. There is also a computed tomography (CT) simulation scanner and treatment planning systems available from multiple vendors. The TDC is staffed by more than 20 full-time personnel, including physicists and dosimetrists with decades of experience in proton therapy treatment. In the TDC environment, hundreds of patient treatments can be simulated in a virtual environment. Prior to the opening of the PPTC in Oklahoma, the radiation therapists, dosimetrists, physicists, and physicians who would actually be treating on-site spent hundreds of hours at the TDC learning on the very equipment they would be using. Various simulations were designed (such as system crashes midtreatment) to prepare the staff for possible treatment situations known to have occurred at other centers.

At the PPTC, the first patient treated was in the room for 37 minutes, which was the "door-to-door" time and included entering the room, patient positioning, setup verification, treatment delivery of three fields, and exiting the room. Within 6 months of opening, the PPTC is capable of treating simple cases (such as prostate) in 15 minutes, intermediate cases (such as intracranial) in 30 minutes, and complex cases (such as craniospinal irradiation and pelvic lymph node irradiation) in 45 minutes. These treatments are delivered using uniform scanning and require field-specific apertures and compensators. Although shorter treatment times do not necessarily imply a higher treatment quality, they do reflect the implementation of a training system that allows for the delivery of proton radiation in a reproducible manner.

■ **WILL PROTON THERAPY PROLIFERATE IN THIS DECADE AS IMRT DID IN THE PREVIOUS DECADE?**

The simple answer to this question is: No.

A concern of many parties, specifically insurers and competing radiation oncology centers that do not have proton therapy access, is if proton therapy will see an exponential growth through this decade much like IMRT rose in the previous decade. The scale and complexity of proton therapy will not allow this to happen. There have been multiple announcements from academic and community practices alike stating their intentions to proton therapy to their patients. Clearly, there is great interest, and hopefully, belief among these centers that protons can improve their ability to deliver care to their patients. But because announcements greatly outnumber actual center openings, there are obstacles to adding proton therapy to a practice.

It is difficult to determine the exact number of conventional radiation therapy facilities in the United States, but this number is probably between 2,200 and 2,500 and there are probably 4,000 to 4,500 EBRT rooms operating (3,4). As of June 2010, there are seven operational proton therapy centers and less than 20 operational rooms. There are three facilities under construction (ProCure Chicago, Hampton University, and ProCure New Jersey). Less than 0.5% of all radiation delivery in this country can be done with proton therapy. Protons, unlike IMRT, require a significant capital investment and purchasing an FDA-approved proton therapy system in the United States is difficult. Newer companies are attempting to develop smaller, single-room systems; but as of July 2010, none of these compact solutions have been FDA-approved.

■ **WHAT WILL BE THE IMPACT OF FOR-PROFIT COMPANIES IN PROTON THERAPY?**

Proton therapy projects are very complex, from many perspectives. Financially, it is very difficult for even the nation's largest cancer centers to underwrite 100% of the costs of a proton therapy center. Nearly all of this country's operating academically affiliated centers were financed with some type of funding from outside that particular university.

The Burr Proton Center at the MGH was partially funded through grants from the National Cancer Institute (NCI). MD Anderson funded its proton center through a public-private partnership that included an investment bank, a health care facilities company, public-employee pension systems, and manufacturers of both medical imaging systems and radiation therapy equipment (5). The University of Florida Proton Therapy Institute (UFPTI) was funded, in part, with $19 million from the city of Jacksonville, $11 million from the state of Florida, and $70 million in bonds (6). To finance the PPTC Oklahoma, a finance model was created that included physician investment, hospital investment, and the acquisition of debt from foreign banks. The underlying theme in this is simple: creating a proton center that does not have stakeholders outside the realm of radiation oncology, regardless of for-profit/not-for-profit status, is difficult, if not impossible. Recognizing this, it is important to build a center in which medical decisions are made by the radiation oncologists who actually work at the center. In the PPTC model, we were able to achieve this. Although ProCure manages day-to-day facility operations, all clinical decisions are made by the radiation oncologists who staff the center.

■ **CAN COMMUNITY-BASED PRACTICES CONTRIBUTE TO RESEARCH?**

It may be surprising to learn that currently there is no umbrella group for proton therapy-based research in the United States, despite all centers sharing a great interest in developing proton therapy protocols, which will be multi-institutional. The MGH and MD Anderson have a joint grant from the NCI and thus have a few opened studies between those two institutions. In our center, we opened a proton registry study before the first patient being treated and to date, more than 96% of patients have chosen to enroll. This study will allow us to follow patients in a prospective

manner and report outcomes. All patients are treated according to practice guidelines. Our center is a member of the Proton Collaborative Group (PCG), a nonprofit entity designed to facilitate multi-institutional proton studies. PCG, which is open to all proton centers who wish to join, will begin enrollment in 2011 to site-specific protocols. Within PCG, there are currently seven protocols that have been agreed upon and will open in summer 2010. There are several other concepts being discussed by the different disease subcommittees. It is our center's hope to have all patients enrolled on specific protocols when they become available. Until then, all patients will be offered enrollment on the registry study.

■ **CAN COMMUNITY-BASED PRACTICES TREAT RARE AND COMPLICATED CASES SUCH AS PEDIATRICS?**

Proton therapy is recognized by many as a preferred radiation modality over traditional x-ray therapy in the treatment of pediatric cancer patients. Our group felt as though it was critical to be able to treat pediatric patients at the PPTC. Being community-based initially posed some challenges.

Two keys to building any pediatric proton therapy practice are to: (a) develop a close working relationship with a pediatric hospital and (b) have anesthesia services available.

While the PPTC Oklahoma City is partnered with a leading Oklahoma-based hospital system, this institution does not have a pediatric oncology service. Fortunately, there was a well-established pediatric oncology group at a large free-standing children's hospital, which is nearby, and a working relationship was quickly established. Currently, all children, including those from out-of-town, are seen by the pediatric oncology team at the children's hospital before and during radiation therapy at the proton center, whether or not they are receiving chemotherapy. Their case is also reviewed by the multidisciplinary team, which includes radiation oncologists from the PPTC, at children's hospital prior to treatment.

For patients who will require daily sedation, our center works with an anesthesia group, which has several pediatric fellowship-trained members. By using experienced pediatric anesthesiologists, coupled with the novel table that can be used for both anesthesia and treatment, our center will have ample treatment slots for pediatric patients, including those who require sedation.

■ PROTONS IN THE COMMUNITY-SETTING: LESSONS LEARNED

Our center has been the first center in the country, if not the world, on several fronts regarding proton therapy:

1. The first to use exclusively uniform scanning for delivery
2. The first to use the MedCom VeriSuite on-board image registration software
3. The first to use custom-built table for combined pediatric sedation and treatment
4. One of the first to use robotic positioning (versus traditional tables)
5. One of the first to use an entirely electronic patient treatment record

The decision to use only uniform scanning and not to commission passive scattering (PS) (at this time) was based on several factors, including being better prepared to incorporate pencil beam scanning (scheduled for 2011). Uniform scanning is similar to PS in that both delivery modes will require apertures and compensators. Uniform scanning is distinct from PS in that a second scattering foil is not required, and magnets are used instead to spread the beam out in the plane perpendicular to the axis. This allows for greater field sizes to be treated to a greater depth. The beam penumbra is also less with uniform scanning than with PS, by approximately 30% (Figure 1). But because the dose deposition is done in layers, tumor

motion along the beam axis is a potential factor. To account for this, patients in whom there may be tumor motion along the beam axis undergo 4-D CT simulation. Tumor motion is evaluated on a case-by-case basis and this is labor intensive. The potential interlayer uncertainties have led to a delay in treating select sites, particularly peripheral lung lesions, until this issue can be better understood. Medial tumors, near the mediastinum and hilum have not demonstrated an unreasonable uncertainty in the patients we have evaluated. Uniform scanning has significant advantages to a PS-based treatment system. The large field size and superior depth of penetration make it feasible to treat new disease sites. Earlier in 2010, our center treated a man with anal canal cancer using protons combined with chemotherapy. We believe this to be the first time protons have been used for this disease site. The treatment volumes were per RTOG 0529, and no compromised to target coverage was made. By using proton therapy over IMRT, the small bowel dose and bladder dose were decreased by 60% and 40%, respectively (Figure 2). This will be a site of future investigation at our center. The sharper penumbra allows for superior dose distributions for prostate cancer, particularly at the prostate-rectal interface. Previous reports with PS protons versus IMRT have already shown a 59% decrease in rectal dose when using PS protons.

Proton therapy suffers from a lack of OBI tools that match those found with linear accelerators. This gap is closing, however. Currently, most proton centers in the United States use a 2D to 2D registration system for daily image guidance. In these systems, usually orthogonal setup films are taken at, or near, cardinal angles and then matched the radiation therapists manually to the digitally reconstructed radiograph (DRR). The MedCom VeriSuite program functions in a manner similar to BrainLab or Cyberknife, in that it reconstructs the CT data set to create a DRR that will match the daily port films. Although this may seem like an intuitive approach to daily image guidance, the implementation of this new software has required many hours of work both at the TDC in Indiana

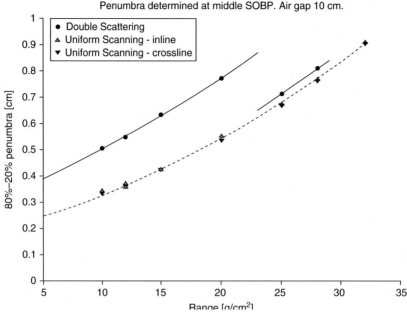

FIGURE 1
Double scattering and uniform scanning at UFPTI. Courtesy of Roelf Slopsema, UFPTI.

as well as at the PPTC in Oklahoma to fully integrate into the daily clinic workflow.

A potential advantage to a community-based proton therapy practice working with a for-profit company that focuses only on proton therapy is the development and implementation of tools to aid in the delivery of proton therapy. Our group believed that we needed to be able to offer proton therapy to children in a standard as high as any academic center. We also wanted to be able to do this in a more efficient manner with respect to room time. In partnering with ProCure, we were able to develop an anesthesia table that would facilitate the treatment of patients requiring daily anesthesia.

This table is a standard K-Vue table (already being used clinically at several proton therapy centers), which has anesthesia equipment mounted at its caudal end (Figures 3 and 4). Thus, this single table can be used during the daily procure of sedation plus treatment from the beginning (when the child is sedated) to the middle (when the child is being treated) to the end (when the child is being recovered). This table has been FDA-approved and will be used starting in September 2010. In our center, the patient will undergo sedation outside the treatment room in an anesthesia bay. The anesthesia table, when not "coupled" to the robotic arm, will sit atop a Stryker trolley. Once the child is sedated, he/she can be transported into the treatment room. All the rooms in the PPTC use a robotic arm for patient positioning, versus a fixed table, which would be permanently fixed into the floor of the room. This robotic arm is accurate and capable of handling payload of up to 200 kg. It has the added advantage of being able to mate to multiple different immobilization devices, including a traditional treatment table, a treatment chair, and the anesthesia table. The robotic arm can "pick up"

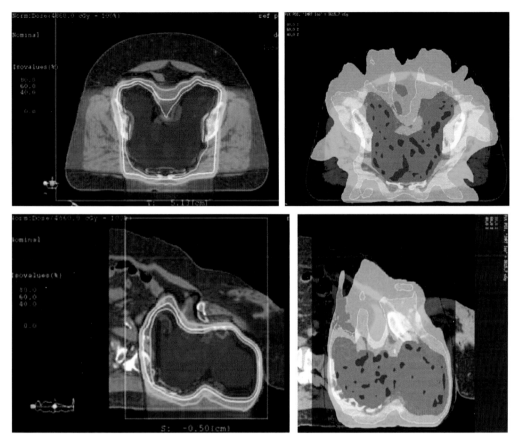

FIGURE 2
Anal canal cancer: proton therapy versus IMRT.

the anesthesia/treatment table using "pin docking." The child will already be in the general treatment position, but final patient position will be established and verified at this stage. Once the patient position is checked and approved, treatment will be delivered. Once the treatment is complete, the anesthesia/treatment table can be placed back onto the Stryker cart and decoupled from the robotic arm. The time required for both coupling and uncoupling from the robotic arm is 90 seconds. Recovery is done outside the room. Using the combination of the anesthesia table with the robotic arm, anesthesia treatments can be significantly streamlined.

■ CONCLUSIONS

Proton therapy is now being delivered in the community, but only in very controlled environments, and is being delivered well. The PPTC Oklahoma City has all of the capabilities of any proton center in a university setting and most of the same missions. While there is a commitment to outside stakeholders, there is a greater commitment to research and innovation. All medical decisions are made by treating physicians. The goal is to keep these tenants in place as more centers, both academic- and community-based, incorporate proton therapy into

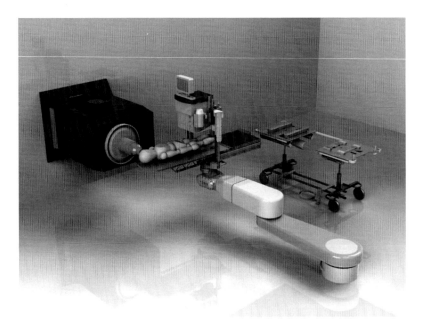

FIGURE 3
The anesthesia unit can be safely brought over the patient as needed.

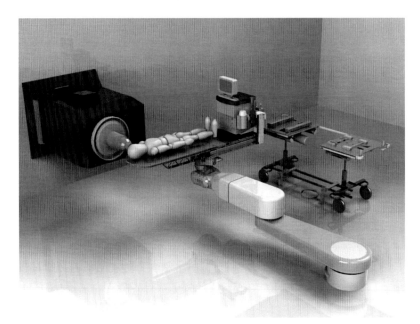

FIGURE 4
The anesthesia unit is returned to the caudal end of the table for treatment.

their practices. The expansion of "big iron" proton centers in the next 10 years will be very limited, because of challenges in financing these centers and building them. If compact single-room systems can be built and approved by FDA, then there will be additional proton capacity in this country. But even if this to occur, it is doubtful that the production of these systems would approach even a fraction of the potential demand.

■ **REFERENCES**

1. Slater JD. Clinical applications of proton radiation treatment at Loma Linda University: review of a fifteen-year experience. *Technol Cancer Res Treat*. 2006;5(2):81–89.

2. MacDonald SM, DeLaney TF, Loeffler JS. Proton beam radiation therapy. *Cancer Invest*. 2006;24(2):199–208.

3. Ballas LK, Elkin EB, Schrag D, Minsky BD, Bach PB. Radiation therapy facilities in the United States. *Int J Radiat Oncol Biol Phys*. 2006;66(4):1204–1211.

4. Owen JB, Coia LR, Hanks GE. Recent patterns of growth in radiation therapy facilities in the United States: a patterns of care study report. *Int J Radiat Oncol Biol Phys*. 1992;24(5):983–986.

5. Rosenthal ET. Proton beam radiation therapy: balancing evidence-based use with the bottom line (part 4 of a multipart investigation). *Oncol Times*. 2010;32(9):28–30.

6. Mendenhall NP. The University of Florida Proton Therapy Institute: An Update. PTCOG 45. October 7, 2006.

Index

Note: Page references followed by "*f*" and "*t*" denote figures and tables, respectively.